The Hospital Guide to Contemporary Utilization Review

Third Edition

Stefani Daniels, RN, MSNA, ACM, CMAC
Ronald L. Hirsch, MD, FACP, CHCQM, CHRI

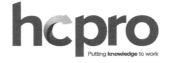

Putting **knowledge** to work

The Hospital Guide to Contemporary Utilization Review, Third Edition is published by HCPro, a division of Simplify Compliance LLC.

ISBN: 978-1-64535-138-2
Product Code: HCCUR3

HCPro provides information resources for the healthcare industry.

HCPro is not affiliated in any way with The Joint Commission, which owns the JCAHO and Joint Commission trademarks.

Stefani Daniels, RN, MSNA, ACM, CMAC, Author
Ronald L. Hirsch, MD, FACP, CHCQM, CHRI, Author

Advice given is general. Readers should consult professional counsel for specific legal, ethical, or clinical questions.

Arrangements can be made for quantity discounts. For more information, contact:

HCPro
100 Winners Circle, Suite 300
Brentwood, TN 37027
Telephone: 800-650-6787 or 781-639-1872
Fax: 800-639-8511
E-mail: *customerservice@hcpro.com*

Visit HCPro online at *www.hcpro.com* and *www.hcmarketplace.com*

Table of Contents

About the Authors

Stefani Daniels, RN, MSNA, ACM, CMAC

Stefani Daniels, RN, MSNA, ACM, CMAC, is founder and senior advisor of Phoenix Medical Management, Inc., a boutique consulting company dedicated exclusively to hospital case management. She is a graduate of Villanova University and has held academic appointments at Columbia University, University of Pennsylvania, and Nova Southeastern School of Business and Entrepreneurship. She began her hospital experience as a critical care nurse back in the dark ages but spent most of her career in the executive suite of hospitals in New York, Pennsylvania, and Florida. She is a member of the editorial board of Lippincott's *Professional Case Management* journal, the coauthor of the popular text *The Leader's Guide to Hospital Case Management,* and a contributing author to the 2nd and 3rd editions of CMSA's *Core Curriculum for Case Managers.* In addition, while in slow retirement mode, Daniels remains a panel member of several webcast groups, including Appeal Academy's Finally Friday and RAC Monitor's Talk Ten Tuesday, when she isn't skiing in Vermont or relaxing on a Fort Lauderdale beach.

Ronald L. Hirsch, MD, FACP, CHCQM, CHRI

Ronald L. Hirsch, MD, FACP, CHCQM, CHRI, is vice president of R1 RCM in Chicago. Hirsch was the medical director of case management at Sherman Hospital in Elgin, Illinois. He is a member of the American Case Management Association, a member of the American College of Physician Advisors, and a fellow of the American College of Physicians. Hirsch serves as an advisory board member for NAHRI.

Preface

by Reggie Allen, MBA, RN

Utilization review (UR) practices still involve prospective, concurrent, and retrospective reviewing of how healthcare resources are used and managed to secure payment for those services. The adage of "no money, no mission" still applies to support a sustainable healthcare delivery system. What has changed over time is the growing importance of these practices, the lessons learned, and the need for better planning based on data.

The advance of electronic medical records offering timely information through various means has not delivered on the hope that much of UR could be automated with physician documentation readily available for claims and reviews. Reviews increasingly require specific knowledge of the information needed and the communication skills required to customize input to each insurer. Knowledgeable reviewers are even more critical now as care delivery is under intense scrutiny. Keeping up with changes in community standards of care, evidence-based protocols, and insurer requirements needs a team of experts to justify and optimize payment for healthcare services.

One major lesson learned is the role of the hospitalist or attending physician extending beyond ordering tests, making diagnoses, and providing medical or surgical treatment. They have now become a significant part of hospital reimbursement. In both concurrent and retrospective medical reviews, physicians employed by insurers often require insurer and hospital physician-to-physician reviews. As treatments and procedures evolve, so does the need for written documentation and rationale for each service. Since insurers still require physicians to document the need for all services, including the level of care, traditional medical record documentation often fails to capture or sufficiently nuance relevant clinical information. To quickly resolve requests for services or claims, insurance companies have found that talking to a treating physician can give needed information for quick coverage decision-making. A challenge lies in ensuring the hospital physician representative is aware of the requirements for a successful negotiation. UR staff, including nurse and social worker experts, no longer work independently. They are now thrust into a team model, with each providing relevant information to direct a successful discussion between the two physicians.

In addition to the changes in UR practices and the team approach with direct physician involvement, perhaps the greatest need is incorporating data, including predictive analytics, and the ability to understand and use this information. Healthcare medical record documentation coupled with administrative and utilization data provides a rich source of information that can be analyzed by informaticists sitting alongside medical experts who ask the right questions and clarify results in medical and operational terms. This is also used to enhance physician engagement in the UR process to see aggregated results of their input and action.

The specialty of UR has become even more critical in the business of healthcare. Dr. Hirsch and Ms. Daniels capture the full scope of knowledge that the successful UR team must have to help guide the revenue cycle team and the hospitalists toward economic success as the face of healthcare continues to evolve. Insurance is a finance scheme intended to increase the benefit to shareholders by reducing the cost of care, often through denial of payment. Insurers do not deny care. They take credit for the care provided in their utilization statistics even if they deny paying a claim for that service. UR addresses this policy and is increasingly important in keeping a hospital solvent.

Reggie Allen, MBA, RN, serves the mission of CHRISTUS Health as chief operating officer of CHRISTUS Spohn Hospital Corpus Christi - Shoreline and Memorial. Having received national and state-level recognition for his work in resource management and clinical operations, he has demonstrated his business acumen through successful implementation of care management, utilization management, case management, revenue cycle, clinical appeals, compliance with federal and state regulations, clinical documentation improvement, and implementation of quality improvement processes in both clinical and business arenas. He has a Six Sigma Green Belt and incorporates quality improvement tools in all his redesigns of clinical operations. He is a member of the American Case Management Association (ACMA) and has served on the editorial board.

Introduction

by *Juliet B. Ugarte Hopkins, MD, CHCQM-PHYADV, FABQAURP*

I'm going to be honest—most of the time, I have no idea why there are multiple editions of a book. Usually the "updates" are minimal or inconsequential. At the end of the day, the umpteenth edition doesn't have much insight beyond what was provided in the first.

Not so here, my friends!

The Hospital Guide to Contemporary Utilization Review was in 2015, and continues to be in 2021, a source of guidance and direction every physician advisor (PA) and other leader in utilization review, case management, and revenue cycle can rely on. Given the nature of the topic and the ever-changing landscape of the field, this updated resource is critical as the payer environment continues to shift to value-based payment models.

While the title of this book includes "utilization review," the focus of our work is morphing into the concept of resource utilization. Instead of case/utilization managers and PAs reviewing decisions made and plans set into place for hospitalized patients, why not attempt to bring the providers themselves into the fold by fostering some element of understanding of hospital resource utilization? "I'm only interested in the medical care of the patient" is no longer a valid statement when there are so many options to consider regarding appropriate care. We are well past the point in medicine where there is a single medication to treat a condition or a single standard of care to evaluate a patient's constellation of presenting signs and symptoms. As physicians and other providers have an escalating array of options available to them, even more effort should be put into understanding how each impacts the patient not only medically but financially, in some cases. If we expect patients to trust us as clinicians when it comes to their physical and psychological health, shouldn't that same trust extend to their financial health? We have moved beyond a black-and-white manner of devising a care plan where there is one path to follow and it is what it is. With so many shades of gray, we have arrived at a moment where physicians simply can't remain ignorant to the financial side of medicine for their patients' sake.

"All I want to do is care for my patients" is a phrase I have heard multiple times when engaging clinicians in discussion about patient status, whether a procedure is necessary for a no-longer-symptomatic individual, or if another night in the hospital is required. We have to insist upon some thought being put into these "business of medicine" concepts, because hospital closures continue to be on the rise. If we don't all pay attention to protecting the hospital from shutting its doors, how will we care for the patients, then? Payment models, regulatory requirements, misuse or overuse of hospital resources—these all come into play when considering hospitals' and health systems' ability to continue providing care to their communities.

I am proud of the continued effort the authors have put into educating and engaging hospital leaders, and I implore you, the reader, not to keep this valuable information to yourself. Chip away at the "I didn't go to medical/nursing school for this" mentality. Build collaborative partnerships between hospital departments while breaking down those traditional silos. It's time to use what you learn here and devise a manner to disseminate it to your providers and the rest of the care team.

Juliet B. Ugarte Hopkins, MD, CHCQM-PHYADV, FABQAURP, is physician advisor for case management, utilization, and clinical documentation at ProHealth Care in Waukesha, Wisconsin. She is a pediatric hospitalist and president of the American College of Physician Advisors. Ugarte Hopkins is certified in healthcare quality and management by the American Board of Quality Assurance and Utilization Review Physicians.

CHAPTER 1

The Origins and Evolution
of Utilization Review

Introduction

It will take years to measure the financial impact on America's hospitals that accompanied the COVID-19 pandemic. While census and operating costs soared with repeated surges of COVID-19 patients, there is ample evidence that the suspension of elective procedures and the drop in nonurgent patient volumes in most states led to an abrupt decline in hospital revenues as patients postponed care due to fear of contracting COVID-19 in the hospital and to stop the spread of the virus.

Although some federal and state rules were relaxed or waived during the pandemic and hospitals got a 20% Medicare payment increase for patients diagnosed with COVID-19, hospital leaders retained their ongoing responsibility to monitor quality and performance, to use resources wisely and appropriately, and to monitor costs associated with the care provided. As of this writing, vaccination against the virus is rapidly spreading across the globe, and it is hoped that the business of healthcare will shortly resume its natural trajectory.

That trajectory, boosted by growing evidence that value-based care (VBC) is economically desirable, will bring hospital leaders back to the table to consider how new payment models and new delivery care models will affect hospital activities in general and utilization review (UR) in particular.

The escalating costs of healthcare in the United States remain the driving force in federal efforts to reduce expenses, while maintaining attractive profit margins drives insurance companies toward the same goals. Similarly, nonprofit hospitals must show a profit margin to invest in modernizing infrastructure or expanding community services. Cost containment is on everyone's mind and will continue to take center stage as the pandemic loosens its grip on the nation's hospital system.

Historically, the emphasis on cost containment has added to the growth of case management programs in many hospitals because case managers were positioned as promoters of the hospital's cost containment strategy. However, as cost containment initiatives have escalated with the rapid introduction of new rules and regulations regarding payment, an inherent conflict has developed: Can the case manager simultaneously be a patient advocate who facilitates care coordination and promotes quality care while also effectively serving as a system agent who is instrumental in controlling costs through the organization's UR program? Because of those payment rules and regulations, which seem to change daily, and the expected expansion of value-based payment models for both federal and commercial payers, hospitals are recognizing that UR activities more properly fall under revenue cycle than care coordination and should be a specialty that stands on its own. As a result, we are seeing a gradual and expanded shift of the UR function from its historical position within a case management program to a new position within the division of finance.

Many argue that the UR process can be tedious and intimidating. Working with the insurance companies on behalf of the patient, the physician, and the hospital can be a frustrating exercise that pits providers against payers. The medical staff may be frustrated by the payer reviewers and don't understand why their medical judgment is being questioned when all they want to do is ensure the patient's well-being. Physicians grumble about what they see as intrusions and challenges from the hospital's UR specialists, clinical documentation integrity specialists, case managers, medical directors, physician advisors, the government, and the insurance companies. Physicians may not necessarily believe that good documentation is a cornerstone of good care. In their siege mentality, they are privately—and sometimes publicly—annoyed when they perceive that someone else is questioning their professional judgment.

Despite the medical staff's aversion to UR activities, UR remains a critical part of the healthcare process because it is essentially an audit of physician documentation, providing a type of internal check and balance that supports patient care. Without a crystal ball, payers and regulators who are looking over the physician's shoulder and overseeing the hospital's compliance processes depend upon that documentation to monitor and evaluate the appropriateness and medical necessity of a treatment, test, procedure, or hospitalization.

UR has come a long way since the early days when physician and nurse reviewers relied solely on clinical experience to make decisions. Today, federal rules and regulations, payer contracts and provider manuals, and the growing expectations of a value-based environment go a long way toward standardizing the review process. A new perspective has emerged that patient advocacy and cost containment are not mutually exclusive.

A History Lesson

As new UR specialists enter the field every year, knowledge of utilization review's evolutionary trajectory will help newcomers better understand its source and its decades-long challenges. As currently structured, the American healthcare industry is a publicly and privately funded patchwork of fragmented systems and programs. Insured Americans are covered by both public and private health insurance, with a majority covered by private insurance plans through their employers, which was an accident of history as employers tried to lure GIs returning from World War II by offering paid health insurance as a recruitment perk. Government-funded programs, such as Medicaid and Medicare, provide healthcare coverage to some vulnerable population groups. The government also publicly funds coverage through Indian Health Services and the military. However, and despite implementation of the Affordable Care Act in 2010, 12.1% of Americans remained uninsured as of 2019 (CDC, 2021).

Medicare and Medicaid

With the signing of H.R. 6675 in 1965, President Lyndon B. Johnson authorized Title XVIII of the Social Security Act to provide health insurance to almost all Americans age 65 or older via the Medicare program. Part A, which was referred to as hospital insurance, was funded by a payroll tax paid by employees, employers, and the self-employed. It had no premiums, and when it was established, there was a $40 annual deductible. Part B was a voluntary program open to citizens of all ages who paid a monthly premium of $3, which was estimated to be enough to fund 50% of Part B costs (with federal revenues covering the remainder). Both programs sought to fill the gaps created by private insurance, which did not offer coverage to high-risk, elderly Americans or to low-income individuals.

Before Medicare and Medicaid, which was enacted as Title XIX, the two-way relationship between the physician and the patient determined which acute care services the patient would receive. If patients had hospital insurance and paid their premiums, they would receive services, and the insurer would reimburse the patient or pay the hospital directly. After the introduction of Medicare and Medicaid in 1965, the two-way relationship between the physician and the patient became a three-sided triangle where the insurer contracted not only with the patient but also with the physicians and the hospitals. As entities statutorily responsible for the appropriate use of taxpayer funds, Medicare and Medicaid assumed the right to monitor the reasonableness and appropriateness of the services being provided. Soon after, by virtue of the contracts signed by the physicians and the hospitals, the insurance companies demanded the same right to monitor services.

Medicare parts

But because financing for each part comes from different sources, CMS has limited ability to shift money from one part to another. As services move from inpatient to outpatient, and as the use of observation services increases, CMS is forced to make payment adjustments on each side. Currently, Medicare coverage works as follows:

Part A: Medicare Part A covers inpatient hospital care, including care provided by short-term acute care hospitals, inpatient rehabilitation hospitals, inpatient psychiatric hospitals, long-term acute care hospitals, skilled nursing facilities (SNF), some home healthcare, and hospice.

Part B: Medicare Part B covers outpatient hospital care, including emergency department (ED) visits, outpatient surgery, outpatient hospital stays with observation services, outpatient testing (such as imaging and laboratory testing), physician professional fees in both the outpatient and inpatient settings, ambulance care, durable medical equipment, some home healthcare, and select medications.

Part C: Also known as Medicare Advantage (MA), Part C plans are offered by private companies that are paid a capitated, per member, per month amount from Medicare to provide care to their enrollees. Unfortunately, there is a lot of confusion among senior populations who succumb to the misinformation and sly advertising geared to mislead potential buyers. Generally, these enrollees find out that they actually enrolled in a Medicare alternative, not regular Medicare, only when hospital care is needed. Part C plans are required to provide care equivalent to benefits available from Medicare Parts A and B, but the Part C plan can limit the contracted providers who provide that care. Part C plans also are permitted to offer extra benefits such as eye care, dental care, and health club memberships. UR professionals should also note that many beneficiaries don't realize that Part C benefits are typically community based, which means they may have to pay out-of-network costs if nonemergent care is provided outside the beneficiary's enrollment location.

Part D: Medicare Part D is the prescription drug benefit. Most Part D benefits are administered by a pharmacy benefit manager (PBM) and offer reduced out-of-pocket costs to patients who use in-network pharmacies and mail-order prescription fulfillment.

Medicare benefits and coverage rules do not always appear straightforward to beneficiaries. For example, coverage for annual doctor visits demonstrate how confusing Medicare benefits can be to some beneficiaries. Federal law prohibits regular Medicare from paying for annual physicals, and patients who get them may be on the hook for the entire amount. But beneficiaries pay nothing for an "annual wellness visit," which is intended "to develop or update a personalized prevention plan and perform a health risk assessment" (CMS, 2021).

Coverage for routine vaccines is another common point of confusion for beneficiaries. Medicare Part B covers some routine vaccinations, such as influenza vaccination and pneumococcal vaccination. It also covers tetanus vaccinations if administered after an injury and hepatitis B vaccinations in medium- and high-risk individuals. But the shingles vaccine, hepatitis B vaccination in low-risk individuals, and Tdap (tetanus, diphtheria, and acellular pertussis) vaccination are covered by Part D. Physicians can administer and bill for vaccines covered by Part B just as they bill for their professional services, but most physicians are not able to bill Part D directly for the vaccinations that the patient's Part D plan covers. As a result, the physician must bill through an intermediary or refer the patient to a pharmacy that is able to administer the vaccine and directly bill the Part D plan. Note, however, that the ongoing efforts by state, local, and federal government to vaccinate the entire United States population against COVID-19 is being completely underwritten by the federal government.

National and local coverage determinations

Part B of Title XVIII of the Social Security Act provides supplementary medical insurance for certain Medicare beneficiaries, specifying which healthcare items or services Medicare will cover. Those items or services are regularly published as National Coverage Determinations (NCD) and describe under what circumstances a test or procedure will be considered reasonable and necessary (and, therefore, payable by Medicare). Consider these NCDs as the federal policy and procedure manual for payment. They are not a standard of care or best practice medical intervention but rather can be thought of as the payer's requirement for coverage and payment. A claim submitted for a test or procedure that has an NCD must be submitted with an associated ICD-10-CM code or narrative diagnosis justifying the medical necessity.

On a local level, Medicare contractors are authorized by CMS to develop Local Coverage Determinations (LCD) for tests and procedures commonly used in their respective jurisdictions. Each LCD is accompanied by an explanation of the coverage requirements; however, payment may be denied if the pertinent medical documentation supporting the requirements does not accompany the claim. Coverage policies are always based on medical necessity and are specific to an item or service. They also define the specific diagnosis for which the item or service is covered.

LCDs may vary from jurisdiction to jurisdiction because they are local. For example, Palmetto GBA (the MAC for Part A and Part B claims in Alabama, Georgia, and Tennessee [Jurisdiction J] and North Carolina, South Carolina, Virginia, and West Virginia [Jurisdiction M]) publishes LCDs specific to each state and identifies under what conditions a procedure, test, or a piece of medical equipment will be eligible for payment. For expeditious claim processing, it is in the best interest of the revenue cycle team and providers to familiarize themselves with the information in these NCDs and LCDs about what medical documentation is required for coverage. The Medicare Coverage Database can be found at *https://www.cms.gov/medicare-coverage-database/new-search/search.aspx.*

Escalating costs after Medicare introduction

Almost immediately following the July 1, 1966, implementation of Medicare, the program's expenditures exceeded the original estimates and continued to accelerate rapidly due to rising costs and the slow and steady increase in the number of beneficiaries (see Figure 1.1). The same increase in Medicare and Medicaid costs was also noted on the commercial side. By 2019, healthcare spending reached $3.8 trillion, or $11,582 per person, and accounted for 17.7% of the nation's gross domestic product (CMS, 2019). The costs of hospital care reached $1.2 trillion in 2019 and, according to CMS "nonprice factors, such as the use and intensity of services, contributed to this steeper growth compared to previous years." When someone asks why this country is in a healthcare crisis, point to the fact that when 17.7% of the GDP—roughly interpreted for the layman as 17.7 cents of every $1—goes to a single commodity, there is less available for other government expenditures, and thus discretionary spending is reduced, schools lay off teachers, roads and bridges don't get fixed, and libraries close.

There are three key drivers that account for the world-leading health spending in the United States: prices, resource utilization, and administrative costs. There are high prices associated with everything from drugs, medical supplies, imaging, and medical devices (Anderson, 2003). At the local level, greater utilization of resources plays an important role and payers, including Medicare and Medicaid, are placing utilization of services under greater scrutiny than ever. Doctors and hospital personnel regularly complain that providing services to patients has become a bureaucratic mess and that they are spending more time on administrative tasks such as calling and writing letters to convince payers to approve coverage or pay claims. This bureaucratic work itself has a cost for both provider and payer organizations. A recent report states that the United States pays nearly $2,500 per capita on administrative costs by insurers and providers, compared to Canada, which pays $551 per capita (Himmelstein, 2020). Taken together, it appears that the United States does more for patients during hospital stays and doctor visits, they're charged more for the service, or both. Any national or state attempt to regulate prices would be met with resistance from all those who directly benefit from high prices, including physicians, hospitals, pharmaceutical companies, and pretty much every other provider of healthcare in the United States.

■ Figure 1.1

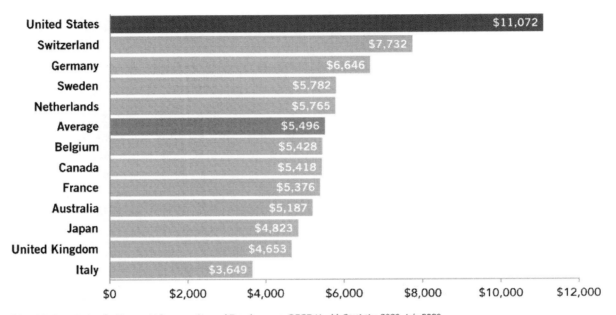

United States per capita healthcare spending

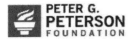 U.S. per capita healthcare spending is almost twice the average of other wealthy countries

HEALTHCARE COSTS PER CAPITA (DOLLARS)

United States	$11,072
Switzerland	$7,732
Germany	$6,646
Sweden	$5,782
Netherlands	$5,765
Average	$5,496
Belgium	$5,428
Canada	$5,418
France	$5,376
Australia	$5,187
Japan	$4,823
United Kingdom	$4,653
Italy	$3,649

SOURCE: Organisation for Economic Co-operation and Development, *OECD Health Statistics 2020,* July 2020.
NOTES: The five countries with the largest economies and those with both an above median GDP and GDP per capita, relative to all OECD countries, were included. Average does not include the U.S. Data are for 2019. Chart uses purchasing power parities to convert data into U.S. dollars.
© 2020 Peter G. Peterson Foundation   PGPF.ORG

Source: Peter G. Peterson Foundation, *https://www.pgpf.org/.*

Concurrent with the introduction of Medicare and Medicaid, private commercial insurers began to take a harder look at ways to curb increasing healthcare costs and introduced the concept of "medical necessity" into their contracts. As one article on medical necessity noted, "The vagueness of the term served providers and insurance companies well because it provided flexibility needed to make discrete coverage decisions" (Bergthold, 1995). This meant that a physician could order a service based on medical necessity in their professional judgment, but the insurer could then deny payment based on their own interpretation of medical necessity for the same service.

The rapid escalation of Medicare and Medicaid costs was generally attributed to three causes: general inflation, an increase in the volume of beneficiaries, and increased intensity of services.

It was the latter category—intensity of services—that accounted for expenses associated with the following:

- New technology
- New and more costly pharmaceuticals

- An increase in the use of selected services
- The use of more costly care even when less costly care is available
- The misuse or overuse of services

These were major cost drivers, and soon after Medicare and Medicaid costs began to escalate, states adopted regulations with different definitions of medical necessity largely based on accepted medical practice at the time. Several states subsequently added cost-effectiveness to their criteria for determining medical necessity.

The federal government made further regulatory and legislative efforts to gain better control over expenses, and in 1969, "Congress created a new system for controlling services financed by Medicare and Medicaid. The original Medicare law had required hospitals to set up committees of their medical staffs to review whether services were actually necessary. But these UR committees, as they were called, had no formal criteria for evaluation, no power to deny payment, and no incentive to be effective" (Starr, 1982).

Trajectory of peer review

Persuaded by the American Medical Association in 1972 to let physicians monitor other physicians, the federal government enacted Public Law 92-603, which included an amendment for the creation of physician-controlled, regional professional standard review organizations (PSRO) to monitor the quality and cost of medical services performed under Medicare and Medicaid. The PSRO was a system of UR committees run by medical organizations and based on peer review. The PSRO Committee on Finance believed the following at the time:

> Medicine, as a profession, should accept the task of advising the individual physician where his pattern of practice indicates that he is over-utilizing hospital or nursing home services, over-treating his patients, or performing unnecessary surgery ... Government should not have to review medical determinations unless the medical profession evidences an unwillingness to properly assume the task.
> (U.S. Senate Committee on Finance, 1974)

However, the PSROs turned out to be a pricey venture and disappointed federal policymakers. They did not succeed in curbing costs, and there is no evidence in the medical literature—or based on our personal experiences—that the organized medical community showed any real concern for monitoring resource utilization or decreasing costs. Therefore, the government was left to regulate the medical community, because as Senator Wallace Bennett said in a speech on the PSROs, "Where organized medicine is unwilling or unable to assume the responsibilities of a PSRO, or where performance of a particular organization is only pro forma or token ... the Secretary [of Department of Health, Education and Welfare, a precursor to HHS] would arrange for the designation of another private or public organization or agency which has the professional competence to undertake the necessary functions" (U.S. Senate Committee on Finance, 1974).

This failure of the organized medical community to monitor their peers haunts them today. Had they fulfilled their obligation to oversee the use of medical resources through peer review when they were given the chance, perhaps the subsequent proliferation of rules and regulations with which we now have to contend could have been avoided. Congress allowed the PSRO structures to sunset, and in 1982, as part of the Tax Equity and Fiscal Responsibility Act PL 97-248, professional review organizations (PRO) replaced the PSRO.

Medical decisions that had been the exclusive domain of the physician and patient were now going to be evaluated by an external reviewer who was accountable to the CMS program. The PROs assumed binding review for hospital services in accordance with *Conditions of Participation (CoP)* as written in 42 *CFR*

§482.30 to ensure that healthcare services provided under Medicare and Medicaid were "medically necessary, conformed to appropriate professional standards, and were delivered in the most efficient and economical manner possible." In 2002, the PROs were renamed Quality Improvement Organizations, and in August 2014, they morphed into two separate programs: Beneficiary and Family-Centered Care Contractors and the Quality Improvement Network.

Similarly, the private insurance companies, not to be outdone by the federal government, determined that they too must closely monitor resource utilization to hold true to the fundamental law of insurance: The payments to the insurer over time must cover the average person's claims and the cost of running the company and leave room for the firm's profits. With published profit margin of 3% in 2019 and net earnings of $23 billion, the profitability of the health insurance industry has never been better (National Association of Insurance Companies, 2019).

Terminology: Is It Utilization Review or Utilization Management?

Over the years, the terms UR and utilization management (UM) began to be used synonymously, which created confusion among hospital stakeholders. No consistent definition distinguishes one term from the other. However, in the real world of hospital operations, there are subtle differences between UR and UM, and each implies different obligations.

Overall, it's best to think of UM as a term to describe the full spectrum of strategies and initiatives that a hospital leadership team has put in place to contain costs, improve operating efficiency, and ensure appropriate use of hospital resources held in trust for the care of the community it serves. UR, on the other hand, is a subset of UM and specifically refers to the tools and methodologies that hospitals and payers use to ensure that hospital level of care is necessary and appropriate for the circumstances presented by the patient.

While some definitions of UR include monitoring of resources being used or prescribed in the care of a hospitalized patient, it is rare for a UR specialist to question specific medical decisions and rarer still for the medical staff to self-review behaviors to identify opportunities to reduce resource utilization. On those occasions when a preauthorization for a hospital service is required by the commercial insurer, the UR specialist is usually the first line of communication with the payer to advocate for the patient to get approval for the services prescribed.

UM initiatives can be prospective, concurrent, or retrospective activities that focus on resource use relative to patient outcomes and delivery of care efficiencies. To orient your organization regarding the differences between UM and UR, consider using the RIGHT rule: That is, UM consists of all the activities that are in place to ensure that the patient gets the right care, in the right place, at the right time, every time! Under new payment models, hospital executives continue to work to maximize efficiency and reduce costs associated with excessive, redundant, or wasteful resource utilization, and UM initiatives will undoubtedly increase to reduce costs per case as penetration of risk contracts increase. Yet the distinction remains confusing to many hospital associates who stubbornly equate it with UR.

The broad category of UM initiatives intended to drive efficiency and reduce avoidable costs rely upon a rigorous focus on performance outcomes throughout the hospital or healthcare system and may include the following:

- Examining triage processes, Emergency Medical Treatment and Labor Act compliance, and use of emergency services
- Shifting level of service assessment activities to points of entry
- Preauthorizing outpatient services
- Monitoring of imaging services
- Monitoring of pharmaceutical usage
- Handling antimicrobial stewardship
- Promoting adherence to nationally recognized blood product indications
- Promoting use of evidence-based guidelines
- Ensuring timeliness of delivery of care processes
- Identifying patient flow bottlenecks and throughput barriers
- Noticing delays in transitions of care
- Avoiding low value and serial interventions

For example, the chief operating officer may initiate a UM project in collaboration with the radiology department to monitor the use of imaging technologies. Radiology may have mechanisms in place to concurrently screen for the appropriateness of the ordered test in relation to the patient's current medical condition, comorbidities, and the expressed intent of the test. Thus, if a physician orders CT scans with and without contrast, a radiologist would review the need for the patient to undergo both scans. If the radiologist finds that the physician's clinical question may be answered by just one scan, he or she would contact the physician for a clarification order. If concurrent monitoring is not feasible, retrospective resource utilization audits on the use of CT scans may be undertaken by the UR committee.

Likewise, if a physician prescribes a costly medication when a less costly one is available and appropriate for the expressed need, the pharmacy director may call the prescribing physician to discuss alternative pharmaceuticals. In each of these cases, a peer-to-peer conversation between the prescribing physician and the physician advisor (PA) might take place to discuss more appropriate and cost-effective options. In today's healthcare world, the quickly developing sophistication of electronic decision support systems makes it possible to conduct the screening process electronically through the use of electronic health record (EHR)–embedded decision support tools.

An example of UM geared toward improving efficiency may include hospital preparations for VBC and population health by assigning case managers to specific populations of patients and following them through the entire continuum of care to minimize gaps in communication, improve clinical information sharing, and avoid duplication or redundancies in resource utilization. Although it's often a challenge to implement in large facilities, regionalization of hospitalists is also a key efficiency component that can get executive teams thinking about how best to meet desired quality and financial goals within the context of a practical infrastructure. Hospital leaders may achieve greater efficiency and improve patient throughput if, for example, they objectively examine the costs associated with the absence of clinical services on the weekends or the rework that must be done in the absence of a front-end UR process. In these cases, just consider the volume of payer denials resulting from "warehousing" patients over the weekend or the costs of back-end fixes that must be made to correct eligibility for inpatient or outpatient services.

UR versus resource management initiatives

As described, UM is the overarching description for all strategies and initiatives used to monitor the appropriate use of hospital-owned resources. UR is a major component of UM, but so are the other initiatives summarized above, which might be categorized as resource management or resource utilization initiatives to differentiate it from the formal—and quite prescriptive—UR activities. Despite the different designations, UR and resource management/resource utilization are related and warrant further discussion to make it clear to our readers.

Utilization review is the process that uses medical documentation to evaluate the patient's clinical status at a specific point in time to establish suitability for acute care services. A nationally recognized criteria set, such as Hearst's MCG Care Guidelines or Change Healthcare's InterQual®, is often used as a guide to help UR specialists assess the safest and most clinically appropriate level of care, but close review of medical documentation is required to determine whether the level of care requires hospitalization and whether care is anticipated to cross two midnights for Medicare beneficiaries. This distinction is very important, as there are still UR specialists who daily confront physicians with the mantra that "Your patient doesn't meet criteria." Medicare has clearly stated that "It is not necessary for a beneficiary to meet an inpatient 'level of care,' as may be defined by a commercial screening tool, in order for Part A payment to be appropriate. In addition, meeting an inpatient 'level of care,' as may be defined by a commercial screening tool, does not make Part A payment appropriate in the absence of an expected length of stay of 2 or more midnights or documented medical necessity for hospital level of care" (CMS, 2014). The content of the admission medical documentation in combination with the guidance offered by the criteria sets is vital to determine an accurate status for the patient as inpatient, outpatient (with observation), or outpatient in a bed (a courtesy distinction with separate billing implications). UR decisions should not be based on criteria alone; they must be based on a combination of criteria and whether the documentation of the patient's current clinical status at the time of the admission supports medical necessity for hospital care. The presence of the former does not mean that the latter is sufficient. Because medical necessity is often based on documentation that has already been written, review of the documentation is a *retrospective process* (except in the ED, where it is a *concurrent process*).

■ Figure 1.2

Utilization review activities

- Prospective reviews of medical necessity are generally reserved for patients scheduled for elective procedures, transfers from other facilities or outpatient areas within an organization, or requests for direct admissions.

- Concurrent reviews of medical necessity are predominantly reserved for the ED, where real-time conversations between the emergency physician, admitting physician, and UR specialists can result in decisions that best meet the patient's immediate needs. In addition to assessing medical necessity, concurrent reviews provide the opportunity to encourage accurate documentation of the patient's clinical condition, influence use of a medical protocol for selected diagnoses, and identify any present-on-admission indicators.

- Retrospective reviews to determine the appropriateness of continuing an acute level of care are retrospective activities heavily dependent on the content and completeness of medical documentation during the patient's length of stay.

Resource management/resource utilization, on the other hand, can be a prospective, concurrent, or retrospective process intended to avoid unwanted events from occurring in the first place. Resource management is what CMS means when it states in the *CoP* that review is required "with respect to the medical necessity of … professional services furnished, including drugs and biologicals" (42 *CFR* §482.30(c)(iii)). Resource utilization reviews may be prospective when evaluating pre-procedure/pre-surgical clearance requirements, concurrent when an antibiotic is being prescribed that is not listed on the culture and sensitivity report, or retrospective when radiology audits the use of CT scans. Concurrent resource management is an essential part of the real-time advocacy responsibilities of a case manager, the patient's nurse, or even the medical director of the lab, imaging department, or pharmacy. Retrospective processes, including monitoring trends and patterns of resource utilization over time, are generally part of the UR committee's duty to identify opportunities to rein in excessive or duplicative use of hospital services.

Rationale for hospital utilization review and resource management

In the past, cost containment efforts by hospital leaders focused primarily on the traditional areas of supplies and labor. Supply costs were most frequently managed by negotiating lower prices and more advantageous contracts, standardizing supply choices, and engaging physicians in supply chain initiatives. Labor costs were addressed through staffing reductions, cutting overtime and agency costs, reducing retirement contributions, and revisiting employee health benefits. However, unsustainable economic trends make it clear that hospital leaders need to do more, and some executives are taking cost management to the next level by reducing controllable expenses.

One method of reducing controllable expenses is implementation of payment models that involve financial risk to provider organizations that fail to manage costs and quality. The pressure to shift to more complex and financially risky payment models is increasing and is already in place in many settings. CMS' risk-based payment models, such as the Medicare Shared Savings Program (MSSP), appear to have helped shift participating accountable care organizations (ACO) to more fiscally sustainable models. For example, in 2012, 94% of all ACOs participating in the MSSP were on the no-risk track. That number dropped to 59% in 2021 as providers learned how to rein in avoidable costs and gain a greater share of savings (CMS, 21 July 2021). Among medical practices caring for capitated populations during the COVID-19 pandemic, net revenue increased even though patients avoided nonessential visits, as the practice still received their payment. Hospital leaders should not wait for legislation to change what they do and must move beyond the industry's burning platform and start taking resource management seriously. It represents a final opportunity to reduce costs and improve quality.

In an era of healthcare reform, the long-term success of organizations requires leaders to shed reactive, tactical approaches in favor of deliberate, well-planned cost reductions. The C-suite must undertake organizational excellence initiatives through resource management and alignment between cost and quality. Hospital leaders are also putting value back into value management by using diagnosis and service benchmarking to identify areas of quality concern and link those areas to financial data, thereby giving proof to the medical staff that there is a need for change. Meanwhile, leaders are looking to resource management and UR to find better ways to deliver quality, safety, and service at much lower cost to remain competitive and to thrive under new payment models.

The Fiduciary Responsibilities of the Board

Today's healthcare industry looks different than healthcare systems from 20 years ago. The hospital has changed from being a strictly inpatient sick care facility to being a community healthcare delivery system. This was borne out by the hospital response to the community during the COVID-19 pandemic. Healthcare and the rules that govern it are constantly changing, and boards are slowly adapting so they are better able to respond to those changes. Although it is true that each board can be considered unique, every board—whether the directors oversee a large academic teaching facility, small critical access hospital, for-profit corporation, or nonprofit institution—benefits from conscientiously observing sound governance and fiduciary oversight. While there are many factors that distinguish for-profit and nonprofit boards, both types must be sure to act in the best interest of the organization and their community.

Hospital boards must work to ensure that the following are true:

- Operating plans exist
- Accurate financial statements are prepared and distributed
- Financial resources are appropriately safeguarded and allocated to achieve near- and long-term organizational goals and objectives
- Management's actions are in the best interest of stakeholders
- Policies and procedures encouraging legal and ethical compliance are in place
- The hospital operates in a fiscally sound manner, with mechanisms in place to keep it fiscally sound

Although there are several differences between public, not-for-profit government-owned hospitals, private nonprofit hospitals, and private for-profit hospitals, board members for each type are legally responsible for ensuring that the hospital is compliant with all applicable laws and regulations and that safe, quality care is available and provided to all patients. Boards differ greatly from management, but both recognize that achieving high value for patients is the overarching goal of the system. High-impact boards whose members are most engaged in the business of sound governance go beyond ensuring compliance, reviewing financial reports, and assessing portfolio diversification: They also analyze what drives value. When the National Quality Forum issued *Hospital Governing Boards and Quality of Care: A Call to Responsibility* (National Quality Forum, 2005), it was strongly suggested that "hospital governing boards become actively engaged in quality improvement" to demonstrate the relationship between governance and quality of care. Working closely with subject matter specialists, today's nonprofit hospital boards will recommend appropriate quality measures and targets to the executive team as well as to the committees on quality and safety. The board should debate alternative strategies, pay close attention to the development of quality measures and reporting requirements, analyze leading indicators of quality, and be schooled on quality, safety, and cost management issues, challenges, and opportunities. The authors of a 2007 publication cosponsored by the Office of Inspector General and the American Health Lawyers Association suggest that governing boards play a vital role in monitoring and improving hospital care to ensure that it is safe, beneficial, patient-centered, timely, cost-efficient, and equitable. The pursuit of "reasonable inquiry" is essential to execute these boards' fiduciary obligations (Callender, Hastings, Hemsley, Morris, & Peregrine, 2007).

A New Marketplace Creates a New Perspective

There are as many definitions of UR as there are insurance companies, professional societies, and healthcare organizations. The most common definition comes from URAC—formerly the Utilization Review Accreditation Commission—a nonprofit accreditation agency that promotes review standards and guidelines for payers and third-party administrators. URAC defines UR as "the process where organizations determine whether health care is medically necessary for a patient or an insured individual." According to the Institute of Medicine, UR is a "set of techniques used by or on behalf of purchasers of health benefits to manage health care costs by influencing patient care decision-making through case-by-case assessments of the appropriateness of care prior to its provision" (Field & Gray, 1989). The process can be concurrent, as it usually is in the ED, or prospective, as it is for elective procedures. But in general, UR within the hospital industry is considered to be a retrospective assessment of the necessity and appropriateness of the allocation of acute care resources based on the physician's documentation of the patient's need for those services.

No matter what you call them, the processes used to evaluate the reasonableness and appropriateness of a medical intervention prescribed by physicians are, by their very nature, challenging for anyone committed to advocating for the patient, the hospital, or the community. Although some organizations have been operating with closed medical staffs for decades and have consistently demonstrated thoughtful resource stewardship, many hospital cultures are not prepared to take the necessary steps to safeguard the use of the facility and the services it offers for patients qualifying for acute level of care. However, as you shall see throughout this book, the hospital industry will be forced to make significant changes in the way it delivers care if it wants to be financially successful in the rapidly changing healthcare environment.

UM activities—both UR and resource management—are no longer perfunctory activities; both are critical economic factors for the hospital's prosperity as the dynamics of the marketplace change and new delivery-of-care and payment models are introduced. The UR specialist role continues to evolve and will continue to grow. UR specialists will be integral to revenue cycle activities and to helping their facilities succeed financially. This book is intended to promote that growth by sharing insights, information, and best practices about UR and resource management to help the reader question past assumptions, prompt discussions, and generate new ideas.

References

Anderson, G. F., Reinhardt, U.E., Hussey, P.S., and Petrosyan, V. (2003). It's the prices, stupid: Why the United States is so different from other countries. *Health Affairs, 22*(3). Retrieved from *https://www. healthaffairs.org/doi/10.1377/hlthaff.22.3.89.*

Bergthold, L. A. (1995). Medical necessity: Do we need it? *Health Affairs, 14*(4). Retrieved from *https://www. healthaffairs.org/doi/full/10.1377/hlthaff.14.4.180.*

Callender, A. N., Hastings, D. A., Hemsley, M. C., Morris, L., & Peregrine, M. W. (2007). Corporate Responsibility and Health Care Quality: A Resource for Health Care Boards of Directors. Washington D.C.: OIG. Retrieved from *https://oig.hhs.gov/fraud/docs/complianceguidance/corporateresponsibilityfinal%20 9-4-07.pdf.*

Centers for Disease Control and Prevention. (CDC). (2021). FastStats—Health insurance coverage. Retrieved from *https://www.cdc.gov/nchs/fastats/health-insurance.htm.*

Centers for Medicare & Medicaid Services. (CMS). (March 2014). Reviewing hospital claims for patient status: Admissions on or after October 1, 2013. Retrieved from *https://www.cms.gov/Research-Statistics-*

Data-and-Systems/Monitoring-Programs/Medicare-FFS-Compliance-Programs/Medical-Review/Downloads/ReviewingHospitalClaimsforAdmissionforPosting03122014.pdf.

CMS. (2019). National health expenditures. Retrieved from *https://www.cms.gov/files/document/highlights.pdf.*

CMS. (July 21, 2021). Medicare Shared Savings Program fast facts. Retrieved from *https://www.cms.gov/Medicare/Medicare-Fee-for-Service-Payment/sharedsavingsprogram/program-data.*

CMS. (2021). Medicare Wellness Visits February 2021 updates. Retrieved from *https://www.cms.gov/Outreach-and-Education/Medicare-Learning-Network-MLN/MLNProducts/preventive-services/medicare-wellness-visits.html.*

Field, M. J., & Gray, B. H. (1989). Should we regulate "utilization management"? *Health Affairs, 8*(4). Retrieved from *https://www.healthaffairs.org/doi/pdf/10.1377/hlthaff.8.4.103.*

Himmelstein, D. U., Campbell, T., and Woolhandler, S. (2020). Health care administrative costs in the United States and Canada, 2017. *Annals of Internal Medicine.* Retrieved from *https://www.acpjournals.org/doi/10.7326/m19-2818.*

National Association of Insurance Companies. 2019 Annual Health Insurance Industry Analysis Report. Retrieved from *https://content.naic.org/sites/default/files/inline-files/2019%20Health%20Industry%20Commentary_0.pdf.*

National Quality Forum (2005). Hospital governing boards and quality of care: A call to responsibility. Trustee. Mar; 58(3):15-8. PMID: 15825939.

Starr, P. (1982). *The Social Transformation of American Medicine.* New York: Basic Books.

U.S. Senate Committee on Finance. (1974). Background Material Relating to Professional Standards Review Organizations. Washington, D.C.: U.S. Government Printing Office. Retrieved from *https://www.finance.senate.gov/imo/media/doc/background.pdf.*

CHAPTER 2

The Regulatory Environment

Healthcare Regulations and Obligations

The healthcare industry is one of the most regulated industries in America. Federal regulations, state and local agencies, and accrediting organizations contribute to what is often described as a burdensome and costly array of mandates that create financial, structural, and procedural requirements for hospitals. Payer contracting activities impose even more requirements, all of which must be tracked, analyzed based on their effect on the organization, and implemented by the responsible parties to maintain compliance. Understanding the nuances of the continuously evolving standards, regulations, and contractual requirements can be a cumbersome task and requires a commitment from the program leader or from one or more team members. This chapter covers some pertinent areas affecting utilization review (UR) practices.

Conditions of Participation

The Department of Health and Human Services (HHS) published the *Conditions of Participation (CoP)* for hospitals in conjunction with the introduction of the Medicare and Medicaid programs in 1966. In order to participate in the Medicare and Medicaid programs, hospitals and healthcare organizations must meet standards set by the *CoP.* The Centers for Medicare & Medicaid Services (CMS) regards these health and safety standards as the foundation for improving quality and protecting the health and safety of beneficiaries. Compliance with the *CoP* is determined by a periodic survey conducted by a state agency on behalf of CMS or a national accrediting organization. The accrediting organization must be approved by CMS and must have standards and a survey process that meets or exceeds Medicare's requirements.

The survey process generally takes place every three years and consists of interviews, document reviews, and observations to validate compliance with each section of the *CoP* in accordance with the survey protocol guidelines. CMS publishes Interpretive Guidelines that serve to define or explain the relevant statute and regulations and do not impose any requirements that are not otherwise set forth in statute or regulation.

Typically, someone in the executive suite receives notification of an impending survey, but hospitalwide preparations are typically organized and tracked through the facility's compliance, quality, or performance improvement director. Each facility has its own process to ensure compliance with the *CoP,* but every program manager or department director is involved. Many organizations also perform mock surveys, either with internal staff or an external agency to assess compliance prior to the actual survey, affording a chance to fix processes and prepare staff.

The survey process is occasionally conducted by a state agency, but it is more often performed by an accrediting agency to which CMS has granted survey authority.

As of this writing, the following organizations have "deemed status" to survey hospitals on behalf of CMS:

- Healthcare Facilities Accreditation Program (previously the accreditation program of the American Osteopathic Association)
- Center for Improvement in Healthcare Quality
- Det Norske Veritas Healthcare
- The Joint Commission

Although this text will concentrate on utilization review, note that the *CoP* include requirements related to discharge planning, nursing services, pharmacy services, medical record services, the medical staff, and other areas that may overlap with the work of the UR professional. Because the UR process is all about documentation, each of these roles and services may affect or be affected by UR (see Chapter 5 for discussion of the UR process). For example, the UR specialist may consult with the patient's nurse or a case manager to gain insight about the patient's condition and weigh it against the physician's documentation. If the documentation does not support the patient's actual condition as described by the nurse, a conversation with the physician may be warranted. Similarly, if the documentation does not include evidence that supports further need for an acute level of care, the UR specialist may bring the matter to the nurse, case manager, or physician and suggest expedited discharge or documentation that justifies a continued acute care stay.

The *CoP* for UR are found in the *Code of Federal Regulations (CFR)* at 42 *CFR* §482.30. All UR departments must comply with these regulations. However, the statutes are written to provide some flexibility, thus permitting each facility to establish a practical process of review that best fits its character (see Figure 2.1).

■ Figure 2.1

Text of 42 *CFR* §482.30 *Condition of Participation:* Utilization Review

The hospital must have in effect a utilization review (UR) plan that provides for review of services furnished by the institution and by members of the medical staff to patients entitled to benefits under the Medicare and Medicaid programs.

(a) *Applicability.* The provisions of this section apply except in either of the following circumstances:

(1) A Utilization and Quality Control Quality Improvement Organization (QIO) has assumed binding review for the hospital.

(2) CMS has determined that the UR procedures established by the State under title XIX of the Act are superior to the procedures required in this section, and has required hospitals in that State to meet the UR plan requirements under §§456.50 through 456.245 of this chapter.

(b) *Standard: Composition of utilization review committee.* A UR committee consisting of two or more practitioners must carry out the UR function. At least two of the members of the committee must be doctors of medicine or osteopathy. The other members may be any of the other types of practitioners specified in § 482.12(c)(1).

(1) Except as specified in paragraphs (b) (2) and (3) of this section, the UR committee must be one of the following:

(i) A staff committee of the institution;

Text of 42 CFR §482.30 *Condition of Participation:* Utilization Review (cont.)

(ii) A group outside the institution -

(A) Established by the local medical society and some or all of the hospitals in the locality; or

(B) Established in a manner approved by CMS.

(2) If, because of the small size of the institution, it is impracticable to have a properly functioning staff committee, the UR committee must be established as specified in paragraph (b)(1)(ii) of this section.

(3) The committee's or group's reviews may not be conducted by any individual who -

(i) Has a direct financial interest (for example, an ownership interest) in that hospital; or

(ii) Was professionally involved in the care of the patient whose case is being reviewed.

(c) *Standard: Scope and frequency of review.*

(1) The UR plan must provide for review for Medicare and Medicaid patients with respect to the medical necessity of -

(i) Admissions to the institution;

(ii) The duration of stays; and

(iii) Professional services furnished, including drugs and biologicals.

(2) Review of admissions may be performed before, at, or after hospital admission.

(3) Except as specified in paragraph (e) of this section, reviews may be conducted on a sample basis.

(4) Hospitals that are paid for inpatient hospital services under the prospective payment system set forth in part 412 of this chapter must conduct review of duration of stays and review of professional services as follows:

(i) For duration of stays, these hospitals need review only cases that they reasonably assume to be outlier cases based on extended length of stay, as described in § 412.80(a)(1)(i) of this chapter; and

(ii) For professional services, these hospitals need review only cases that they reasonably assume to be outlier cases based on extraordinarily high costs, as described in § 412.80(a)(1)(ii) of this chapter.

(d) *Standard: Determination regarding admissions or continued stays.*

(1) The determination that an admission or continued stay is not medically necessary -

(i) May be made by one member of the UR committee if the practitioner or practitioners responsible for the care of the patient, as specified of § 482.12(c), concur with the determination or fail to present their views when afforded the opportunity; and

(ii) Must be made by at least two members of the UR committee in all other cases.

(2) Before making a determination that an admission or continued stay is not medically necessary, the UR committee must consult the practitioner or practitioners responsible for the care of the patient, as specified in § 482.12(c), and afford the practitioner or practitioners the opportunity to present their views.

(3) If the committee decides that admission to or continued stay in the hospital is not medically necessary, written notification must be given, no later than 2 days after the determination, to the hospital, the patient, and the practitioner or practitioners responsible for the care of the patient, as specified in § 482.12(c);

(e) *Standard: Extended stay review.*

(1) In hospitals that are not paid under the prospective payment system, the UR committee must make a periodic review, as specified in the UR plan, of each current inpatient receiving hospital services during a continuous period of extended duration. The scheduling of the periodic reviews may -

(i) Be the same for all cases; or

(ii) Differ for different classes of cases.

Text of 42 *CFR* §482.30 *Condition of Participation:* Utilization Review (cont.)

(2) In hospitals paid under the prospective payment system, the UR committee must review all cases reasonably assumed by the hospital to be outlier cases because the extended length of stay exceeds the threshold criteria for the diagnosis, as described in § 412.80(a)(1)(i). The hospital is not required to review an extended stay that does not exceed the outlier threshold for the diagnosis.

(3) The UR committee must make the periodic review no later than 7 days after the day required in the UR plan.

(f) *Standard: Review of professional services.* The committee must review professional services provided, to determine medical necessity and to promote the most efficient use of available health facilities and services.

The preamble to 42 *CFR* §482.30 states, "The hospital must have in effect a utilization review plan that provides for review of services furnished by the institution and by members of the medical staff to patients entitled to benefits under the Medicare and Medicaid programs." Whether the physicians on staff are employed by the hospital or are independent, hospital leadership is obligated to ensure that the services provided to patients are safe, effective, and medically necessary. This is accomplished by developing and implementing a UR plan that speaks to how the hospital will determine the appropriateness and medical necessity of admissions, duration of stays, and the use of professional services. The UR plan and committee will be discussed in detail in Chapter 7.

CMS also publishes the Survey Protocol, Regulations, and Interpretive Guidelines for Hospitals, which are found in Appendix A of the *State Operations Manual* (SOM). These regulatory guidelines provide survey agencies with a narrative description of the elements of the *CoP* and explain how CMS expects the deeming agency to survey the hospital. These narratives are referred to as survey procedures and provide suggestions about which medical records, hospital policies and procedures, and committee minutes should be reviewed. Hospitals are not mandated to follow the suggestions for survey procedures cited in the narratives, but advance knowledge of these suggestions may help the facility and individual departments prioritize internal preparation activities.

CoP change proposals

In 2015, CMS proposed a significant change to the discharge planning *CoP* (CMS-3317-P). This proposal included a requirement that formal discharge planning be performed for all outpatients who receive observation services and for outpatients undergoing surgery with anesthesia or moderate sedation. In early 2018, it was believed that this proposed rule would sunset at the three-year time limit for official action, but in late October 2018 CMS issued a formal extension of timeline for publication of a final rule, noting that exceptional circumstances warranted exceeding the mandated timeline. CMS noted "the development of the final rule requires collaboration with the Department of Health and Human Services' Office of the National Coordinator for Health Information Technology" as justification for the delay (CMS, 2018).

In November 2019, CMS finalized the rule (CMS-3317-F and CMS-3295-F). In this final rule, CMS did not finalize the requirement for formal discharge planning for select outpatients but did add several significant requirements, including offering patients written choice of post-acute providers, including home health, skilled nursing facility, acute rehabilitation, and long-term acute care hospital providers. That list must include all home health providers that serve the area in which the patient resides and that request to be listed by the hospital as available. For the other post-acute providers, the list must include all facilities in the geographic area requested by the patient. CMS also specified that hospitals may not develop a "preferred list of providers" but may designate if any facility offers specialized services that are needed by the patient. As of this writing, CMS has not yet updated the Interpretive Guidelines for Discharge Planning even though the new requirements are in place (CMS, 2019).

With these added requirements, many organizations have begun using electronic methods of offering choice of post-acute providers, with systems designed to be highly customizable, sorting providers by ZIP code, distance, and ratings. The patient and/or patient representative are directed either to a website for the search or offered a portable computer to review the options. These methods do not produce a written copy of the choices offered to the patient, so it is important that there be documentation to support the method used to provide the patient the list and that the process can be reproduced if a surveyor asks to see how the choice is offered.

Although the *CoP* apply specifically to patients whose care is funded by Medicare and Medicaid, they generally apply to all patients who receive care at the hospital. This is a logical way for hospital leaders to handle *CoP* because hospital personnel care for many patients who have no insurance or who will later be determined to be eligible for Medicaid or other patient assistance programs.

Medicare Advantage

Medicare Advantage (MA) plans, also known as Medicare Part C, continue to expand enrollment. Many states are also turning some, if not all, of their Medicaid recipients over to managed care organizations in an attempt to reduce costs and improve coordination of care. Approximately 24 million Medicare beneficiaries (approximately 39% of all Medicare beneficiaries) were enrolled in an MA plan in 2020 (Freed, Damico, and Neuman, 2021). An MA plan is a replacement for traditional Medicare and provides coverage that is equal to or better than Medicare Parts A, B, and often D. MA beneficiaries may appreciate the lower out-of-pocket costs and the additional benefits, but their choice of providers is often limited when they require specialty care, hospitalization, or post-acute care. In addition, it's important to remember that most MA plans are community based. If members need healthcare in an area distant from the geographic enrollment site, they may be required to compensate for out-of-network costs. This is especially relevant if a member lives part-time in a snowbird state such as Arizona or Florida.

Many MA plans also provide benefits, such as vision care, dental care, and health club memberships, that are not available to original Medicare beneficiaries. In early 2018, CMS widened the range of services MA plans can offer to include items such as groceries, air conditioners, grab bars, and even nonskilled care in the home. These additional benefits are intended to improve or maintain beneficiary health.

CMS' *Medicare Managed Care Manual* is a separate policy manual for MA plans. The manual delineates all the compliance, coverage, and payment regulations along with required beneficiary protections. CMS specifies that MA plan enrollees must have access to benefits that are equal to or better than traditional Medicare either by furnishing the services directly, through arrangement, or by paying on behalf of the enrollee. The manual specifies the following:

Several original Medicare covered benefits and services are covered only for specific benefit periods, e.g., inpatient hospital services, skilled nursing facility services, and inpatient psychiatric hospital services. While an MA plan may offer additional coverage as a supplemental benefit, it may not limit the original Medicare coverage. MA plans must provide their enrollees with all basic benefits covered under original

Medicare. Consequently, plans may not impose limitations, waiting periods, or exclusions from coverage due to pre-existing conditions that are not present in original Medicare (CMS, 2016).

As an example of a benefit that is above and beyond the coverage offered by traditional Medicare, many MA plans waive the three-day inpatient stay requirement for patients who require care that can be safely provided in a skilled nursing facility (SNF). Such plans can offer this benefit to their members because the financial responsibility for the SNF stay falls on the MA plan. CMS has also granted many of the pioneer accountable care organizations (ACO) a waiver on the three-day requirement to assess the financial and clinical effects of waiving that requirement. They also incorporated a waiver for the three-day stay requirement starting in year two of the Comprehensive Care for Joint Replacement program and as an option in Models 1, 3, and 4 of the Bundled Payment for Care Improvement programs.

Although the scope of benefits is clearly delineated in the *Medicare Managed Care Manual,* CMS considers MA plans' requirements for UR processes and payments to hospitals to be a contractual issue and does not regulate them. As a result, many MA plans have implemented precertification requirements, established proprietary level of care stratification tools, and hired independent organizations to perform audits of inpatient admissions in a manner similar to that of a Recovery Audit Contractor (RAC)—not to deprive beneficiaries of needed care but rather to avoid paying providers for that care.

If a provider is not contracted with the MA plan, the plan is obligated to follow all Medicare rules. The 2-midnight rule, which will be reviewed in an upcoming chapter, does not apply when determining status for MA patients who are hospitalized at hospitals that are contracted with the MA plan. However, the 2-midnight rule does apply if the hospital is not contracted. MA plans are not bound by the 2-midnight rule when dealing with contracted hospitals because it is considered a contractual issue and the status determination of a hospitalized patient is not related to the care the patient receives. In other words, an MA beneficiary placed as outpatient will receive the same care as an MA beneficiary admitted as inpatient, meeting the requirement that MA beneficiaries receive the same benefits as original Medicare.

UR specialists and physician advisors (PA) spend a great amount of time and effort sorting out the proper status for MA beneficiaries (and other commercial payer beneficiaries). To understand why this confusion occurs, it is important to look back at the early days of Medicare. Medicare divides medical care into two parts, A and B. Funding for each part is separate: Part A is funded by payroll taxes while Part B is supported by funds authorized by Congress and premiums paid by enrollees. Since these are separate funds, the services provided must be separately designated as Part A or Part B services. In general terms, Part A covers inpatient care and Part B covers outpatient care, including outpatient hospital care. Over time, CMS' rules and guidance for defining and differentiating inpatient and outpatient hospital care have evolved. Because the budgets for Parts A and B are separate and both are fixed, CMS must adjust payment rates to keep expenditures separate and carefully account for all services.

On the other hand, MA plans replace Parts A and B. CMS pays the MA plan a monthly amount for every patient to cover all of their inpatient and outpatient care. As a result, the MA plan has a single large bucket of money to spend on all services, and it is up to the MA plan and the provider to negotiate how much every service is paid. That means that the distinction between inpatient and outpatient is, for MA beneficiaries, an artificial one. The financial distinction, however, is very real for the payer and provider organizations. For example, according to the contract between Hospital A and MA Payer B, a four-day inpatient admission for pneumonia is paid as a diagnosis-related group (DRG) at $8,000, but an outpatient admission with observation services is paid at a fixed observation rate of $4,000. This may create a financial incentive for the payer to deny inpatient admission when it does not impact medically necessary care while simultaneously incentivizing the hospital to more aggressively pursue inpatient admission approvals whenever inpatient care is remotely reasonable. On the other hand, if, according to the contract terms, that payer reimbursed observation at a rate of $3,000 per day, a four-day outpatient observation stay would be financially better for the hospital. In an example from a hospital in the southern United States, the hospital's contact with one MA payer paid inpatient surgeries based on a set fee schedule, whereas outpatient surgeries were paid as a percent of charges. A finance executive at the hospital realized that this contract provision meant the payment for the same surgery done as outpatient was significantly more than inpatient. The hospital then stopped trying to get inpatient approval for surgery.

An MA plan's UR staff are generally not aware of the details of each contract with provider organizations. These staff will base admission approvals on the payer's proprietary criteria and may avoid approving inpatient admissions when possible while ensuring that the patient receives the necessary medical care. Such an approach, however, means the plan's UR staff may not realize that in some instances the plan is paying more for outpatient care than it would have paid for inpatient care.

In the absence of practical reform to the current payment system, MA plans will continue to deny inpatient admissions and hospitals will continue to argue for inpatient status. Although this is primarily a financial issue and appropriate, medically necessary care is provided whether the patient is an inpatient or outpatient, the importance of this issue should not be diminished. It must be remembered that hospitals are the ultimate safety net for a community and most provide millions of dollars of uncompensated care that is only partially reimbursed by the government. Hospitals can continue to operate only if their revenue matches or exceeds their expenses. When hospitals close, communities suffer. When medically necessary care is provided to a patient with insurance, the hospital should expect to be paid fairly for that care.

However, not all questions of admission authorization and MA plans are purely financial. For example, if a physician determines their patient would benefit from inpatient rehabilitation and the patient meets CMS' requirements for those services but the MA plan does not authorize the stay, the patient is potentially being deprived of a benefit available to an original Medicare beneficiary. In this case, the patient may file an expedited appeal with the MA plan, or the physician or hospital may obtain an Appointment of Representative form, CMS-1696, and file the expedited appeal on the patient's behalf.

These examples should encourage PAs and UR staff to research these types of MA contractual issues at their organizations. Despite common goals, it is often difficult to establish working relationships with the hospital finance and contract teams. Tracking issues such as these and presenting the data to leadership can often lead to positive outcomes for both the hospital and the patients.

Hierarchical Condition Categories

To understand the cost-conserving tactics used by MA plans, it would be helpful to understand how CMS pays MA plans for their enrolled beneficiaries. Each year, the insurers' demands for information increase as they attempt to feed their huge data warehouses and fulfill their obligations to the Healthcare Effectiveness Data and Information Set (HEDIS), where they must report information used to measure performance and produce the data that allows CMS to risk-stratify MA beneficiaries. UR specialists should also be aware of the concept that CMS uses to pay the MA plans to provide care to enrollees. CMS pays the MA plan a capitated rate, which is a set amount of money per enrollee per month to provide all covered care. That amount is determined by CMS based on a system called Hierarchical Condition Categories (HCC). The HCC system uses patient demographics and a complex system of hierarchical rankings of the patient's documented diagnoses to assign him or her to one or more of 86 HCCs. Each HCC is associated with a risk score. The patient's total risk adjustment factor (RAF) score is then applied to a base monthly payment rate to arrive at the monthly capitation payment that the MA plan will receive for that patient. There are a few exceptions to this capitated rate, such as clinical trial costs and hospice care.

The effects of the social determinants of health on individuals' overall well-being and health risks are being increasingly recognized. Certain ICD-10-CM codes may be assigned to capture a patient's social determinants of health (Z55 to Z65), but these codes are not assigned any risk adjustment in the HCC paradigm. Recently, several payers and the American Medical Association have called for expansion of the appliable codes and incorporation of them as formal risks that would change a patient's RAF score. Addressing the social determinants of health are beyond the scope of this book, but ensuring that the codes for those determinants are captured and placed on the claim is certainly within the realm of the UR team. Social determinants of health affect every aspect of patient care, from their nutritional status leading to slower healing and a longer length of stay to ease in making plans for post-hospital transitions of care for patients with insecure housing.

Each patient's risk score resets back to baseline each year, and all diagnoses must be documented again to be considered in HCCs for that year's scoring. The HCC ramifications on payment are the reason that so many commercial payers prefer using portals to the hospital's electronic health record to capture as many pieces of information as possible: These diagnoses are then used to demonstrate a higher risk score. It may also explain why the volume of medical record requests from MA plans has skyrocketed—especially in physician offices.

Compliance

Compliance with local, state, and federal regulations is the bedrock of a hospital's operations. Although most hospitals have a compliance department and a compliance officer, all hospital employees and medical staff should work to ensure compliance. An in-depth analysis of all regulations related to compliance is beyond the scope of this book, but we will review the major compliance areas here.

The False Claims Act prohibits knowingly submitting or causing another to submit a false claim to the government or knowingly making, using, or causing a false record or statement to get the government to pay a false claim (31 U.S.C. §3729). Many False Claims Act cases are filed by whistleblowers as "qui tam" lawsuits, which means that an employee who has knowledge of the activity—and may have informed the provider's compliance department of their concern without any response—initiates the lawsuit and becomes eligible for a percentage of any settlement or judgment.

The Anti-Kickback Statute prohibits the exchange (or offer to exchange) of anything of value in an effort to induce (or reward) the referral of federal healthcare program business (42 U.S.C. §1320a-7b). The most common scenario is a physician employed or contracted by the hospital who is paid based on the volume of services referred to the hospital.

The Physician Self-Referral Law, or Stark Law, prohibits a physician from making referrals for certain designated health services payable by Medicare to an entity with whom that entity (or an immediate family member) has a financial relationship (ownership, investment, or compensation), unless a safe harbor applies (42 U.S.C. §1395nn). An example of a prohibited referral would be a physician referring Medicare patients to a home care agency owned by his or her spouse.

UR specialists and PAs are often the first to become aware of a potential compliance issue, whether it's a question about a hospital policy, such as guidelines on the determination of the proper admission status of a patient, or a physician ordering services that do not meet medical necessity guidelines. The hospital's culture should freely allow consultation with a compliance officer to report and investigate such situations. There are strict regulations regarding hospital self-reporting of compliance issues to the government, and time is of the essence in reporting and investigating such activities. It is worth noting that, in most situations, there is no fraud but rather a lack of adequate documentation or a misinterpretation of a rule.

Regulatory and administrative agencies

CMS reports that 6.3 million inpatients and 25.4 million outpatients were served in 2019 for a total of $138.5 billion and $81 billion, respectively (CMS Fast Facts, 2021). The sheer volume of claims filed on behalf of these beneficiaries demonstrates the need for a variety of agencies to manage claims processes. The estimated dollar amount of improper payment is also staggering. CMS reported that the improper claim payment rate for fiscal year 2020 was 6.27% for Medicare parts A and B, representing about $25.74 billion in improper payments, a 13% decline from 2019. The corresponding rate for Medicaid is 21.36%, representing $86.49 billion in improper payments (CMS, 2020). It is important to note that improper payments do not all constitute fraudulent claims. In many cases, the complexity of the claim process leads to improper claims that are unintentional.

Major contractors tasked with processing claims, auditing claims, and working to reduce the number of improper claims include the following.

Medicare Administrative Contractors (MAC): MACs are private healthcare insurers that have been awarded a geographic jurisdiction to process claims for Medicare Part A and Part B. These claims include facility charges, professional fees, transportation charges, and durable medical equipment charges. The MACs also process all denials by other contractors and manage overpayments and underpayments after notification by the contractor. The MAC also acts as the first level of review—the redetermination—for all denials. MACs conduct audits of claims to ensure that they are accurate, the service was reasonable and necessary, the beneficiary is entitled to the benefit, and the claim is not a duplicate of a previously paid claim. In 2017, CMS adopted the Targeted Probe and Educate claim review process where, instead of auditing all providers, specific providers will be selected for claim review based on an analysis of past claims data.

Qualified Independent Contractors (QIC): CMS tasks QICs with making decisions regarding Medicare claim denials at the second level of the Medicare appeals process, known as the reconsideration stage.

Quality Improvement Organizations (QIO): The QIOs were restructured in 2014 into two separate types. The Beneficiary and Family-Centered (BFCC) QIO contractors review quality of care and respond to beneficiary complaints. The Quality Innovation Network (QIN) QIOs work with providers on quality improvement projects. Prior to this restructuring, there was one QIO per state. This system was not ideal because in this setup, it was possible that a QIO working with a provider on a quality improvement initiative would have to evaluate a beneficiary complaint against this same provider, which obviously interferes with objectivity. In late 2015, CMS tasked the BFCC-QIOs with reviews of the short-stay inpatient admissions for compliance with the 2-midnight rule. The BFCC-QIO is best known as the organization that a Medicare beneficiary would call if he or she wished to appeal his or her hospital discharge, per the Important Message from Medicare (IMM) notice.

The Comprehensive Error Rate Testing Program (CERT): The CERT program reviews a sample of all Part A and Part B claims to ensure the accuracy of claims submitted by providers and the accuracy of claim processing by the MACs. The results of CERT audits are provided to the MACs to guide their audits and to educate providers on proper billing and documentation.

Unified Program Integrity Contractor (UPIC): UPICs were formed in 2016 to combine the activities of the Zone Program Integrity Contractor, the Medicaid Integrity Contractor, and the Program Safeguard Contractor. The UPIC contractors use a variety of data to focus their program integrity efforts by identifying vulnerabilities; selecting specific providers for review and investigation; referring potential fraud, waste, and abuse cases to law enforcement; and pursuing administrative actions in Medicare and Medicaid.

Payment Error Rate Measurement (PERM) program: The PERM program measures improper payments in Medicaid and the Children's Health Insurance Program and produces error rates for each program.

Supplemental Medical Review Contractor (SMRC): The SMRC performs medical reviews under the direction of CMS, which chooses the provider and/or topic to review. The SMRC evaluates medical records and related documents to determine whether Medicare claims are billed in compliance with coverage, coding, payment, and billing practices.

Recovery Audit Contractor (RAC): The RAC program began in 2005 as a demonstration project in six states and became a nationwide program in 2009 after it reported overpayments amounting in billions of dollars. The RACs receive a percentage of each improper payment they find and report, and each issue audited by the RACs must be approved by CMS. In 2015, CMS made major enhancements to the RAC audit process by lowering the number of records that may be audited in each six-week period, allowing providers 30 days to request a discussion prior to submitting the denial to the MAC for recoupment, limiting patient status reviews to a six-month lookback period, paying the contingency fee on appealed cases only after the denial has been affirmed at the second level of appeal, and more. As of June 2021, there are 179 issues CMS approved for audit by the RACs, including several for "medical necessity and documentation requirements" for cataract removal, bariatric surgery, and total hip arthroplasty.

Risk Adjustment Data Validation (RADV): The RADV contractor performs audits to check the accuracy of the HCC codes submitted by MA plans for payment. Because the RADV audits are audits of the MA plans, most hospital utilization staff will not interact with these contractors. However, medical records may be requested by the plan to help the auditors validate diagnoses that they have submitted to CMS.

Other auditors: CMS also hires contractors to review the auditors' activity to ensure that their audits are accurate. For example, the RAC validation contractor reviews denials from the RACs to ensure that the denial was proper. If the denial is found to be improper, then there is a process allowing the RAC to dispute the decision. If there is a high RAC error rate on denials, the RAC must provide CMS with a corrective action plan, but there is no provision to reverse the improper denial and repay the provider for the payment that was improperly recouped.

The Office of Inspector General (OIG): The OIG, a division within HHS, identifies waste, fraud, and abuse in all of the divisions of HHS, including Medicare, Medicaid, the Food and Drug Administration, the Centers for Disease Control and Prevention, and the National Institutes of Health. The OIG issues routine reports of provider billing audits, establishes and monitors corporate integrity agreements (CIA) with providers who violate federal regulations, and publishes advisory opinions on topics of interest to providers to determine whether these issues would violate any fraud and abuse laws.

As an example of a widely relevant advisory opinion, on October 29, 2015, the OIG indicated that hospitals will not be subject to OIG administrative sanctions if the hospitals discount or waive beneficiary payments for noncovered self-administered medications that the beneficiaries receive in outpatient settings, including observation, that may be covered under Medicare Part D or are subject to the conditions outlined in the memorandum (OIG, 2015). During the COVID-19 public health emergency, the OIG released advisory opinions and guidance on the many nuances of providing testing, care, and vaccination that could potentially be viewed as risk-prone in a nonpublic health emergency. For example, the OIG laid out circumstances where providers could offer rewards or incentives in connection with receiving a vaccination, an activity that is generally prohibited.

The OIG releases its *Work Plan* that details the areas of concentration for its investigative activities, and each month they issue a snapshot report of their findings. Compliance officers, revenue cycle personnel, and UR specialists should become familiar with the format of the OIG's website and subscribe to the agency's *Work Plan* updates to stay informed (recently added and active *Work Plan* items can be found on the *Work Plan* page of the OIG's website at *https://oig.hhs.gov/reports-and-publications/workplan/index.asp*).

The OIG is not intent on reviewing UR activities. Instead, it uses the claim form information to target cases for review. Hospital compliance officers should be aware that it doesn't take many cases for the OIG to establish an unusual pattern or trend. If such a pattern is found, the OIG will extrapolate data obtained from a modest sample of cases to like claims to establish the basis for a demand for repayment, which often results in an overpayment claim in the millions of dollars. A recent example of this can be found in an article Ronald L. Hirsch wrote on the experience of Genesis Medical Center in Davenport, Iowa (Hirsch, 2018).

Of particular interest is the OIG's recent focus on hospital compliance with the Post-Acute Care Transfer Act (PACT) of 1998. This act requires CMS to adjust Medicare payment to hospitals when patients are transferred to another facility. Under Medicare's PACT policies, hospital DRG payments are prorated, or reduced, when a patient is transferred to another hospital or to select post-acute care settings, including home health services depending on the length of stay in comparison to the geometric mean length of stay designated by CMS for the DRG. Specific details on this policy may be found in Chapter 4 of the *Medicare Claims Processing Manual,* Section 40.2.4.

In August 2020, the OIG released a report detailing its audit of Medicare's oversight of PACT compliance. For the audit, the OIG selected a sample of 150 claims from fiscal years 2016 and 2017. Of that sample, the OIG found that Medicare improperly paid 147 claims, resulting in $722,288 in overpayments. These claims should have been paid the graduated per diem rate rather than the full DRG, according to the OIG. Based on those findings, the OIG estimated Medicare improperly paid hospitals $267 million in a two-year period.

As a result, CMS implemented new system edits, and claims with condition codes 43 (home health not within three days of discharge) and 42 (home health not related to inpatient stay) will receive extra scrutiny. Reader, beware!

Reports and resources

Program for Evaluating Payment Patterns Electronic Report (PEPPER)

PEPPER is a type of comparative data report that provides information on hospital-specific Medicare data statistics for discharges vulnerable to improper payments. This data can help identify both potential overpayments as well as potential opportunities for revenue optimization through process improvements. PEPPER was created by TMF Health Quality Institute and is now administered by the RELI Group to prioritize hospital-specific findings and to provide guidance on areas where a hospital may want to focus auditing and monitoring efforts. PEPPER identifies areas of potential overcoding and undercoding as well as areas that may be questionable in terms of medical necessity for admissions. In 2018, PEPPER also added yearly data on Medicare Spending Per Beneficiary to allow hospitals that have not yet started value-based payment programs to compare their spending to other hospitals nationally. In 2020, the percent of total knee arthroplasty performed as inpatient was added to the report. For more information, go to *www.pepperresources.org.*

Medicare Learning Network (MLN)

CMS has developed a wide range of learning resources for providers, including written publications and live and recorded video tools. The most popular publications are *MLN Connect,* a weekly publication with varying topics related to CMS policies and updates, and *MLN Matters,* articles released on an as-needed basis to address coverage, billing, and payment rules for specific provider types. To subscribe to the MLN resources, go to *https://www.cms.gov/Outreach-and-Education/Outreach/FFSProvPartProg/Electronic-Mailing-Lists.*

CMS manuals and transmittals

CMS publishes a series of manuals that are used by providers, contractors, and survey agencies to administer CMS programs. CMS uses the manual to operationalize regulations published in the *Federal Register* and the *CFR.* The manuals are organized based on functional areas including eligibility, entitlement, claims processing, benefit policy, and program integrity. There are currently 20 manuals that can be found at *https://www.cms.gov/Regulations-and-Guidance/Guidance/Manuals/Internet-Only-Manuals-IOMs.* While the laws and regulations are considered the "source of truth," in practicality, most providers use the manuals for daily interpretations.

When CMS makes policy or process changes in their manuals, it publishes a transmittal. The primary purpose of the transmittal is to convey the necessary information to the contractors so that changes can be made to their processes. Reviewing transmittals allows one to be aware of program changes that may affect provider processes. The transmittals can be found at *https://www.cms.gov/regulations-and-guidance/guidance/transmittals.*

Regulatory notifications to beneficiaries

Advance Beneficiary Notice

The Advance Beneficiary Notice of Non-Coverage (ABN) is provided to patients who are going to receive an outpatient service that will not be covered by Medicare and for which the patient will be expected to pay. As the name implies, the ABN must be presented prior to performing the service. In the emergency department, ABNs cannot be presented prior to the Emergency Medical Treatment and Active Labor Act (EMTALA)-mandated medical screening examination. ABNs cannot be given routinely to all patients just in case Medicare does not pay, and each service that would be denied must be listed. Issue this notice as far ahead of the procedure as possible to give patients adequate time to consider their decision about whether to proceed with the procedure and time to contact the ordering provider to determine why a noncovered service is being ordered. In the UR notes, document the time that the form was presented and the time that it was signed. This provides evidence that the patient did not feel they were coerced into signing a document to get a service that they feel is necessary and has been ordered by their provider.

Although many services subject to ABNs are ordered by physicians, ensuring that the ABN is provided and completed is the regulatory responsibility of the entity performing the service. This can create challenges, as the laboratory technician drawing blood for a test ordered by a physician is unlikely to know why the test is not covered. To avoid any payment misunderstandings, the outpatient registration department should establish policies to screen services for medical necessity and coverage. The department should have procedures in place to obtain the proper information from the physician for accurate completion of the ABN before the patient arrives at the hospital.

There are two classes of ABNs designated by CMS: mandatory and optional. Mandatory ABNs are for services that Medicare sometimes covers but may not cover for this individual patient in this specific circumstance. For example, Medicare covers thyroid blood tests when a patient has an established thyroid disease or symptoms that may be related to thyroid disease, but it does not cover testing as part of a routine physical examination. If a patient presents with an order for a thyroid blood test with no indication of a thyroid-related diagnosis on the script, contact the physician to obtain more information—if available—or present an ABN. The financial liability for such a test would be small, but ABNs may also be required for outpatient procedures that can shift financial liability of tens of thousands of dollars, as when a patient is scheduled for outpatient placement of an automatic implanted cardioverter-defibrillator. In this case, if the patient does not meet the criteria set out in the national coverage determination (NCD), an ABN would be given, and the patient would be responsible not only for the cost of the device—which exceeds $20,000— but also for all hospital services, device implantation, and any hospital stay after implantation.

Mandatory ABNs can also be provided to patients who insist on being hospitalized when there is no medical necessity indication, or for patients whom the physician places as outpatient with observation services despite the absence of any hospital-level needs. This commonly occurs when an elderly family member is brought to the hospital because the family no longer wants to or is unable to provide their care. The use of an ABN in these situations should be a last resort provided only after the family is made aware of community resources available to them and it is clear that there are no acute medical issues or concerns about the patient's safety or potential elder abuse. In this case, the patient would be hospitalized as an outpatient, and the hospital would indicate on the ABN that hospital care, including nursing and room and board, are being provided but are not medically necessary. The hospital would obtain an order for observation services, ask the physician to document that the services are not medically necessary, and present the ABN.

Optional ABNs, on the other hand, can be used for services that Medicare never covers, such as cosmetic surgery, routine eye exams, and routine dental care. Using an ABN in this situation provides two benefits: It enables the provider to have written proof that the patient is accepting financial liability and also permits the provider to bill Medicare knowing that it will be denied, which allows the claim to pass on to the secondary insurer, which may cover the charges. If an ABN is not used in these situations, the patient may still be charged. The mechanics of billing a claim that has an ABN are outside the purview of a UR specialist. However, the UR specialist should ensure that the billing staff knows that an ABN was used so they can add the proper modifiers to the claim and establish payment arrangements with the patient.

Hospital Issued Notices of Non-Coverage (HINN)

HINNs are used for inpatient services when it is believed that the services will not be paid by Medicare. CMS has created several types of HINNs to fit the many situations where they may be needed.

The pre-admission/admission HINN, also known as the HINN-1, is one of the most underutilized tools available to the UR specialist. That is because the pre-admission HINN does NOT require concurrence of the attending physician nor the QIOs prior to issuing the notice to the patient. As such, it is best used in the emergency department before the patient is on the patient unit. Pre-admission/admission HINNs are given to patients when the hospital staff feels that inpatient admission is not medically necessary or custodial in nature and is likely to be denied. This situation could also arise when a physician admits a patient for an inpatient surgery and there is inadequate documentation in the medical record to meet the medical necessity requirements, such as with spine surgery where a trial of conservative measures, or contraindication to such, is not documented. It can also be used when a physician is admitting a patient for inpatient surgery and the UR staff determined that the proper status is outpatient, but the physician is unwilling to change the status or document his or her rationale for inpatient admission. Status determinations for surgery will be discussed in detail in Chapter 5. As noted, unlike other HINNs, advance physician or QIO concurrence is not required, so it could conceivably be a political hot potato that warrants executive discussion before implementing.

The other common use of the pre-admission HINN is for the patient who insists on being admitted as an inpatient because he or she wants to be able to stay three days to access his or her Part A SNF benefit or has the often-mistaken belief that the financial liability is lower with inpatient admission. Because the pre-admission/admission HINN does not require the concurrence of the admitting physician, admitting the patient and simultaneously presenting the pre-admission HINN gives the patient rights to an immediate appeal by the BFCC-QIO. That makes the BFCC-QIO—rather than the hospital or physician—the bad guy in the eyes of the patient when they rule that inpatient admission is not medically necessary. Note that there are negative implications if a doctor acquiesces to the patient and admits him or her without medical necessity and the patient stays the requisite three inpatient days to gain access to part A SNF benefits. Specifically, the *CFR* requires that the three consecutive days in the hospital be medically necessary, and without that medical necessity determination, the patient has not met the requirements. This may result in a denial of payment for the SNF stay and shifting of the financial obligation of those costs to the beneficiary.

If that situation arises, the following steps are recommended:

1. First, if you want to preserve the organization's relationship with the SNF, inform the SNF that a pre-admission HINN was presented to the patient during the intake process. Doing so will allow the SNF to negotiate with the patient and family about advance payment.

2. Second, the patient and the SNF should be informed, in writing, that if the SNF accepts the patient based on the presumption that he or she qualified for his or her Part A SNF benefit, then the hospital will not be held financially liable if the claim is later denied, because the hospital's UR staff does not feel that the stay was medically necessary.

The HINN 11 is used to notify an inpatient who is hospitalized for a medically necessary reason that a service he or she is scheduled to receive is not medically necessary and the patient will be held financially liable. In other words, the patient needs to be in the hospital, but they do not need this particular service. An example is a patient who is hospitalized for an acute exacerbation of systolic heart failure who asks his or her physician to order an MRI of the spine because he or she has some mild back pain. In this case, the patient requires hospital care for his or her heart failure but does not meet the medical necessity requirements for an MRI. It should be noted that under the DRG payment system, performing and billing the MRI is unlikely to result in any additional revenue to the hospital, but because there are costs associated with performing the service, that expense can be shifted to the patient. If the MRI is performed, the study will be interpreted by a radiologist, and results will be provided to the ordering physician. The professional fees associated with the interpretation of the study are not subject to denial in the way that the facility charges are. Another scenario that also carries a significantly higher financial liability would be if the physician for that same heart failure patient schedules the patient for placement of an implantable cardioverter defibrillator (ICD), where the patient's echocardiogram demonstrates an ejection fraction of 38%, which is above the 35% threshold cited in the NCD. In this case, the presence of the ICD on the claim results in a change in the DRG and a significantly higher payment. If that ICD placement is removed from the claim because of lack of medical necessity, the DRG will change and the payment for the admission will be significantly lower. The signed HINN 11 will allow the hospital to recoup payment from the patient for that unnecessary procedure.

A more common situation where the HINN 11 is *not* appropriate involves a patient who is hospitalized for a medically necessary reason but whose physician orders a test that the patient receives as an inpatient, even though it would be more appropriate and safer to perform the test as an outpatient. This is often referred to as the "while you are here" test. Because there is medical necessity for the test, the patient cannot be held financially liable by issuing a HINN 11. In these cases, the UR specialist and physician advisor should work with the provider to explain that additional tests performed during an inpatient admission add expense for the hospital without any additional revenue and request that the testing be deferred until after discharge. An example would be a patient who is admitted as an inpatient for treatment of heart failure. A CT scan obtained during the admission reveals a thyroid nodule. An ultrasound of this nodule would be indicated to better characterize its nature, but there is no need to perform that scan during this hospital admission; it can be safely performed as outpatient after discharge, without any adverse effects on the patient's health or safety.

There also may be a circumstance where the hospital UR staff determines that a patient's continued stay is not medically necessary, but the physician does not concur and is unwilling to discharge the patient. If this occurs, the physician advisor or a member of the medical staff leadership should first be contacted to review the case and speak with the physician, if appropriate. If, after determining that continuing hospitalization is not medically necessary, the physician will not discharge the patient, then the UR specialist should issue a **HINN 10,** also known as the Notice of Hospital Requested Review. In this case, the HINN 10 notifies the patient that the hospital will be contacting the BFCC-QIO to review the case; no action is needed by the patient.

The HINN 12 is the form that notifies the patient that if they remain in the hospital that they will incur financial liability. If the patient has appealed their discharge to the BFCC-QIO, and the BFCC-QIO has ruled in favor of the hospital, the HINN 12 indicates that the patient will be responsible for costs beginning at noon the next day if they choose to remain in the hospital. In the event that the patient is notified that they are stable enough to be discharged and they have received the follow-up IMM if appropriate and the patient chooses not to appeal to the BFCC-QIO, the patient should be given the HINN 12 at that time and financial liability begins at midnight. It should be noted that while MA patients receive the Important Message from Medicare and have full appeal rights, they do not receive the HINN 12 as do traditional Medicare beneficiaries. If financial liability is to be shifted to the patient, the provider must notify the MA plan and determine how they should notify the patient.

It should be noted that the discharge appeal process does not result in the discharge of the patient; the patient remains under the physician's care in the hospital. However, if the hospital had requested the review, it should lead to the patient questioning the physician about why they are remaining in the hospital and being held financially responsible rather than being discharged.

Since the patient remains as an inpatient in the hospital during and after the appeals process, until the patient agrees to discharge, the hospital medical staff bylaws govern how often the patient must be seen by the physician. If it has been determined that the patient does not have medical necessity for continuing hospital care, the medical necessity for daily physician visits may also be questioned even though they are mandated by the bylaws. Physicians should be cognizant of this regulatory dilemma and proceed accordingly.

Because noncoverage would shift financial liability from the hospital or payer to the patient, these decisions should not be taken lightly. Hospitals cannot bill Medicare for unnecessary or uncovered services, but at the same time, asking the patient to assume the costs has the potential to create political and financial fallout. For example, if a patient was told by a physician that a service will be covered and then receives a notice asking the patient to accept financial liability, confusion and frustration will likely result. That patient may lose confidence in the physician and wonder whether the proposed care was being ordered solely to take advantage of the patient and make money. That patient may also choose to post about their negative experience on social media, go to a local newspaper to complain, or score the hospital and physician poorly on a satisfaction survey. Therefore, ensure that all measures have been taken to resolve the need for a notice of noncoverage prior to its issuance.

The use of ABNs and HINNs is complex and requires strict adherence to the procedures set out by CMS for their use. The chief compliance officer or UR staff should always refer to the beneficiary notice initiative website *(www.cms.gov/Medicare/Medicare-General-Information/BNI/index.html?redirect = /BNI/)* and carefully follow the instructions to use the proper forms there. Contact the BFCC-QIO if there is uncertainty about the applicability of the ABN or HINN in a specific situation. It should also be noted that CMS updates the forms every three years; using an out-of-date form invalidates that form and the patient cannot be held liable if an expired form is used. Since the use of these forms should be infrequent, ensuring that the current form is used is critical.

Important Message from Medicare

Every Medicare patient, including those insured by an MA plan, is given a copy of the IMM within two days of inpatient admission and a second copy within two days of discharge. The IMM spells out the patient's appeal rights, which the patient may exercise if he or she feels that he or she is being discharged too soon. If the patient chooses to exercise that appeal right when the physician discharges the patient and subsequently contacts the BFCC-QIO, the QIO will instruct the hospital to issue a Detailed Notice of Discharge to the patient while the QIO reviews the case. If the QIO renders a decision in favor of discharge, or if the patient elects not to appeal the discharge, the patient should receive the HINN 12, which notifies the patient that he or she will be liable for the cost of care from the time designated on the form, which will either be noon the next day if the QIO ruled in favor of the hospital or at midnight on the day the HINN 12 is issued if the patient elects not to appeal.

Generally, the first copy of the IMM is included in the pack of admission information that every patient (or patient representative) must sign during the inpatient registration process. This can be provided by the registration staff with the availability of UR staff if the patient has a question. Although a verbal explanation is not required by statute as with the Medicare Outpatient Observation Notice, CMS expects providers to ensure that patients understand the content of any notice provided. In many cases, at the time of inpatient admission the patient is confused or incapacitated and delivery to the patient at that time should not be attempted. If delivery is deferred at that time, a clear process should be in place to ensure the IMM is delivered within the next two calendar days.

The provision requiring a second copy of the IMM within two days of discharge is often the most difficult for hospitals to operationalize. It is difficult to anticipate when a patient is going to be discharged, and if an unexpected discharge occurs in the evening or on a weekend, there may not be appropriate staff members present to provide the IMM to the patient. CMS has also expressly forbidden the practice of giving the second copy of the IMM to every patient on a regular basis, such as every Monday, Wednesday, and Friday, just in case they are discharged. It is crucial that hospitals hardwire the second IMM delivery process. This second notice can be a copy of the first signed notice and does not require explanation or signature, so a patient's nurse or other support staff can complete this task if needed. The documentation must simply state that the follow-up copy was provided to the patient.

It should also be noted that if the second copy of the IMM is presented on the day of discharge, the patient should be allowed to stay an additional four hours to decide whether he or she wishes to appeal his or her discharge. If the patient agrees to be discharged, then the patient does not need to stay the full four hours. Finally, because the length of stay for many patients drops as hospital care becomes more efficient, it is important to watch the dates on the IMM. A patient who receives the first copy of the IMM on day two of a hospital stay would not need the second copy unless his or her length of stay exceeds four days.

If a patient has chosen to appeal his or her discharge, the patient will remain inpatient in the hospital during the QIO review of the case. The patient should continue to receive medically necessary care under the direction of the attending physician along with the indicated nursing services. The physician is under no obligation to order services or treatments that the physician has determined to be not medically necessary. The patient should also not receive care that may be medically necessary but can safely be provided after discharge.

The discharge appeal process is occasionally used by patients to accrue the three inpatient days necessary to qualify for a Part A SNF benefit. If a patient's appeal is unsuccessful, then the days spent in the hospital awaiting that appeal decision are not counted toward the three inpatient days because the determination from the BFCC-QIO was that the days were not medically necessary. This issue is not directly addressed in CMS regulations or manuals; it is therefore suggested that when the BFCC-QIO contacts the hospital with the determination, the BFCC-QIO representative be asked if the days count toward Part A SNF qualification and that their response, and identifying information, be recorded in the medical record.

Medicare Outpatient Observation Notice

Required as of March 2017, the Medicare Outpatient Observation Notice (MOON) is mandated for all Medicare and Medicare Advantage patients who receive more than 24 hours of observation services. The MOON was the result of the Notice of Observation Treatment and Implication for Care (NOTICE) Act, passed by Congress and signed by President Obama in 2015 in response to the numerous complaints from beneficiaries of their long hospital stays where they were never admitted as inpatients and therefore had no Part A coverage for their SNF stays. The MOON informs patients that their status is outpatient, that their outpatient days do not count toward the days needed for a covered SNF stay, that their financial liability is under Part B, and that their self-administered drugs are not covered by Part B.

The MOON must be provided to all patients who receive more than 24 hours of observation services, but the form may be given before hour 24. It must be presented by hour 36 or sooner if the patient is discharged or admitted as inpatient. The MOON regulations require that the patient receive an oral explanation of the MOON in addition to signing and receiving a copy of the form itself. Because CMS requires patients who receive more than 24 hours of observation services and are subsequently admitted as inpatient to get both a MOON and an IMM, patients may be confused by the different terms in the forms. Explain that the first midnight they spent in the hospital will not count toward the three inpatient days needed for Part A SNF coverage, and the financial aspects of the MOON will not apply to patients unless they are hospitalized at a critical access hospital, where patient liability is based on a different formula than that used for prospective payment hospitals.

The delivery of the IMM and MOON to all applicable patients is a condition of participation, but it is not a condition of payment. That means that if the proper notice was not delivered to the patient, the claim is still payable. Nevertheless, the hospital should consider a performance improvement project to improve adherence and be able to demonstrate to a surveyor that it is continuing to improve its processes.

The MOON form is a standardized notice and must be given to the observation patient even if the patient is not enrolled in Part B. The form includes all of the informational elements required by the NOTICE Act and is available on the CMS website in both English and Spanish. The first page of the form has an open text field that begins with the following: "You're a hospital outpatient receiving observation services. You are not an inpatient because …."

CMS stated that checkboxes may be used to complete the subsequent section, which contains reasons that the patient is not being admitted as an inpatient, but these reasons must be specific to the patient and based on the clinical rationale. This requirement can be met by having wording such as, "You require hospital care for evaluation and/or treatment of [fill in chief complaint]. It is expected that you will need hospital care for less than two days." The chief complaint can be obtained from the patient's record and entered by clerical staff, thus bypassing the need to involve the physician in an administrative task.

Figure 2.2 is the top portion of the first page of the MOON with some sample language that may be used to simplify the form completion process. CMS states that if checkboxes are used, there must be an area for free text in the event that the provider wishes to provide more detailed information ("other" on the form). This sample also includes language about MA. Because the MA plans are not required to follow the 2-midnight rule and often require hospitals to treat patients as outpatient with observation services for several days, this option informs the patient that the insurer—not the hospital—made the status decision. The goal is to make sure that the patient understands that the hospital is simply following federal rules for Medicare and MA beneficiaries.

■ **Figure 2.2**

Medicare Outpatient Observation Notice

Patient name: **Patient number:**

You're a hospital outpatient receiving observation services. You are not an inpatient because:

☒ According to Medicare rules, we are using this time to complete an evaluation of your _____ [fill in chief complaint] to determine if you need to be admitted or discharged.

☐ We do not anticipate that the care you need right now to care for _____ [fill in chief complaint] will not exceed two midnights in the hospital and according to Medicare rules, that does not qualify for a hospital admission.

☐ Your Medicare Advantage plan has told your doctor to place you in Observation.

☐ Other:

Being an outpatient may affect what you pay in a hospital:

- When you're a hospital outpatient, your observation stay is covered under Medicare Part B.

- For Part B services, you generally pay:
    - A copayment for each outpatient hospital service you get. Part B copayments may vary by type of service.
    - 20% of the Medicare-approved amount for most doctor services after the Part B deductible.

Condition code 44

In 2004, CMS introduced the condition code 44 (CC44) through *MLN Matters SE0622*. This code is used to change to outpatient the status of a patient who was improperly admitted as an inpatient. The CC44 process is often referenced as the change from inpatient to observation, but keep in mind that observation is a service provided to outpatients. This process is intended to be used infrequently and not as a substitute for concurrent review of patients needing hospitalization to determine the correct admission status. It should also not be used for a patient who was properly admitted as an inpatient based on the 2-midnight rule but who subsequently improves faster than expected, a patient who is transferred to another hospital or to hospice, a patient who leaves the hospital against medical advice, or a patient who dies. Once a Medicare patient is formally admitted as an inpatient pursuant to an admission order from a qualified practitioner, the patient's status can be changed to outpatient only by using the CC44 process. Even the physician who wrote the original admission order cannot unilaterally revert the patient's status to outpatient.

A compliant CC44 process has four requirements:

1. The case must be reviewed by a physician member of the UR committee
2. There must be concurrence of the attending physician
3. The patient must still be a patient in the hospital
4. The hospital cannot have already billed for the stay

CMS has clarified that an outsourced physician advisor may not authorize a CC44, as the physician member of the UR committee must be a voting member of the medical staff. There also must be an order to change the status to outpatient; documentation of the concurrence of the attending physician and the UR physician; and written notification to the patient, physician, and hospital of the status change. Once the CC44 process has been completed, the entirety of the patient's stay becomes outpatient. This circumstance is the only one in which CMS allows a retrospective status order. If the patient continues to require hospital care after the status change is made, an order should be obtained for observation services. A compliant way to do this would be to include an order in the chart transcribed by a nurse, stating, "Change status to outpatient, discussed with Dr. Hirsch, UR committee. Both concur that patient does not require inpatient care. Telephone order. Read back. From Dr. Jones, attending physician, by S. Daniels, RN."

The CC44 process, if indicated, should be performed as early as possible in the patient's stay so that observation services can commence, as there must be eight or more hours of medically necessary observation for the hospital to receive payment for that care. Performing the CC44 process later in the stay allows the change to outpatient to be made but does not allow the hospital to collect any revenue for the nursing services and room and board provided to the patient. Although inpatients have immediate appeal rights related to discharge, inpatients have no option to appeal their change from inpatient to outpatient via the CC44 process. There is a federal lawsuit (*Alexander v Azar*, 3:11-cv-1703) seeking to grant immediate appeal rights to Medicare beneficiaries whose status is changed from inpatient to outpatient via the CC44 process. The suit is pending at the time of publication.

CC44 is an example of the complexity of understanding the regulatory hierarchy because different regulatory authorities within HHS say different things regarding this process. A CMS consumer publication entitled "Are You a Hospital Inpatient or Outpatient?" contains the following statement:

> *Your doctor writes an order for you to be admitted as an inpatient, and the hospital later tells you it's changing your hospital status to outpatient. Your doctor must agree, and the hospital must tell you in writing—while you're still a hospital patient before you're discharged—that your hospital status changed.* (CMS, 2014)

However, the actual regulation, 42 *CFR* 482.30(d), states that the patient must be notified in writing within two days. The federal regulation takes precedence over the CMS publication, and therefore notification is required within two days. That said, if the status change must be made while the patient is still in the hospital and readily accessible, there is no logical reason not to provide the written notification at that time.

It should also be noted that the CC44 process described here applies only to traditional Medicare patients. In many instances, other insurers have "required" the use of CC44 when the payer is refusing to approve inpatient admission and requests the provider bill the admission as outpatient. There is a distinct difference between the CMS requirement for the CC44 process to change an inpatient to outpatient and a non-Medicare payer's requirement to use CC44. While the former requires the case be reviewed by a physician member of the UR committee and the other steps followed, the latter simply requires that the billers place the "44" in the condition code section of the claim if an inpatient admission is being billed as outpatient.

Self-denial of inpatient admissions

The UR specialist may be called upon to help review short inpatient stays to determine whether the initial inpatient admission decision was correct. Prior to the 2014 Inpatient Prospective Payment System (IPPS) final rule, if an admission was not medically necessary and the patient should have been cared for as an outpatient, the admission could be self-denied and the hospital could then bill for a limited number of ancillary services that were provided to the patient.

In the 2014 IPPS final rule, CMS gave hospitals the ability to self-deny the inpatient admission and then rebill all eligible services provided during the hospital stay under outpatient Part B (Type of Bill 13X) and inpatient Part B (Type of Bill 12X). This self-denial process must follow the process as described in 42 *CFR* 482.30(d), including review by a physician member of the UR committee, discussion with the attending physician, and notification delivered to the patient, physician, and hospital within two days. The revenue cycle staff typically handles the logistics of the actual self-denial and rebilling processes (refer to *MLN Matters SE1333*). While it is preferable to find inappropriate inpatient admissions during the patient's stay and make the change to outpatient with the CC44 process, the lack of adequate staff on weekends and evenings will occasionally let a short-stay admission slip through the cracks. Most hospitals will review all these Medicare one-day, and often two-day, inpatient admissions for appropriateness of the inpatient admission decision and use the self-denial/rebill process as appropriate.

Commercial Insurance Contracts

Complying with Medicare and Medicaid insurance requirements is an obligation governed by federal and state laws. However, contracts, policies, and provider manuals determine the insurance requirements for the many patients whose care is paid for by nongovernmental sources. The variety of sources for commercial insurance requirements can present challenges to the UR specialist, as UR rules for every patient could differ depending on his or her insurance and that insurer's policies.

For example, one insurer could require the strict use of a commercial tool for determining level of care, whereas another could use the tool as the first step in the process, followed by a secondary review by a physician. Many commercial payers have also added a time element to the status determination decision, requiring all patients whose stay is under 48 or 72 hours to be billed as outpatient, even if commercial criteria for inpatient admission are met. The ability for payers to set these seemingly arbitrary criteria is governed by payer and provider contracts that often specify that "the provider agrees to abide by all payer policies." These contracts are often reviewed and approved by the hospital finance team without input from the UR staff. Additionally, many insurers require notification when one of their patients is hospitalized but will not consider that notification to be an authorization for the hospital stay, meaning that payment for the hospital stay can still be denied. Although CMS and MACs publish coverage determinations and make it the providers' responsibility to determine whether a service is medically necessary, commercial insurers often require precertification of scheduled services, such as advanced imaging, surgery, drug administration, and transfer for post-acute care. This precertification requirement often falls upon the UR specialist, who then must gain access to the clinical information supporting medical necessity to convey that to the insurer.

The commercial health insurance market plays a large role in determining the financial viability of the acute care hospital. But although Medicare's impact on hospital revenue is significant, CMS only pays roughly 70–80 cents on the dollar compared with commercial payers, leaving hospitals scrambling to break even. Because the profits on most Medicare payments are small, hospitals must successfully negotiate with the private sector to make up losses. In the past, hospitals were able to negotiate contracts that paid a percentage of charges, which enabled them to cost-shift their losses from Medicare and Medicaid patients to the commercial insurers. Today, those contracts are few and far between, with most commercial insurers switching to fixed rate payments similar to CMS' DRG methodology. They also may insist on a per diem contract, which will only pay for each approved day with variable rates depending on the patient's location in the hospital. In the case of such contracts, the case manager or UR specialist can be certain that the insurer will require reviews for each day to determine medical necessity for that day and for the patient's location in the hospital, whether it is an intensive care unit or a monitored step-down unit.

Contract negotiators should take advantage of whatever leverage they have to create a win-win arrangement. For example, a small community hospital or critical access hospital may have good leverage since they are usually the only game in town and the payer does not want their member to have to travel many miles just to get a chest x-ray or other outpatient diagnostics. Similarly, a hospital designated as "sole community provider" status presents a great leverage opportunity since they are facilities which are 35 miles or more from another provider and, once again, a payer doesn't want to hear complaints from their members about the distance they have to travel for a CT scan or MRI or even for a minor procedure. Whatever leverage can be exercised during negotiations should be considered.

The new price transparency rules imposed on hospitals have also affected pricing and contracting. While initially hospitals were required to post only their chargemaster, which provided patients with little usable information, as of January 2021 the requirement was expanded to require that prices be posted with their codes (e.g., Current Procedural Terminology® code) and that a list of 300 shoppable services be posted in a consumer-friendly manner. The posted prices must also include the highest and lowest negotiated prices and the price for uninsured patients. The overall effect of this requirement is not clear. Some believe that competing hospitals will have access to proprietary pricing information, which could lead to upward pressure on price negotiations, and others feel this will increase competition and drive prices lower.

MA plans should be treated as commercial payers. UR specialists should remind the chief financial officer, revenue cycle committee chair, or the vice president of finance to make sure that reports generated by finance or information services clearly distinguish between MA beneficiaries and original Medicare beneficiaries. Ensuring this distinction is preserved in reports is critical to tracking MA challenges that should be addressed during contract negotiations. This data is also vital to payer mix reporting. A 50% Medicare payer mix should mean that 50% of patients have original Medicare. It should not mean that 30% is original Medicare and 20% is MA. Combining the data from these populations can complicate any problem-solving discussions among the UR committee. This challenge is especially apparent when looking at observation percentages. Although original Medicare regulations for observation are clear, many MA plans use drastically varying definitions of how long observation can last and when it can be used. Comparing observation rates between hospitals with varying MA patient volumes will provide misleading information and may result in adopting noncompliant policies to fix an observation rate.

As the hospital industry inexorably shifts to a value-based environment that incentivizes providers to provide higher-quality care rather than higher quantity, contracts are changing, too. Fixed rate and per diem payments are still popular, but many hospitals, especially those participating in ACOs, are now entering into capitated contracts in which a fixed payment for each member is paid to the provider each month. Hospitals are also entering into bundled payment contracts, where all costs are combined into a single payment, as well as contracts that are based on clinical and/or financial outcomes. The latter are referred to as risk-based contracts because the providers are at financial risk, depending upon whether they achieve predetermined benchmarks. Upside risk contracts refer to arrangements in which the provider may earn additional revenue for outcome achievements but would not suffer any financial loss if benchmarks were not met. Downside risk contracts refer to payment penalties that are imposed if the provider fails to achieve predetermined outcomes or benchmarks. The majority of insurance companies have publicly stated that they will continue to require value-based contracts.

Physicians often pride themselves on treating patients equally regardless of insurance. But if physicians ignore insurance-specific details, such as out-of-network specialists, nonformulary medications, or a transfer to a SNF that is not part of the insurer's post-acute care network, then "equal" treatment is as far from patient-centered as one can get. The UR specialist, case manager, and discharge planning team must work closely with physicians to prevent issues like these.

Contract terminology

Every contract contains terminology describing the payer's expectation of the provider's cooperation with the payer's UR activities. The wording is typically brief and provides a general overview, leaving more specific language for the provider manual. Contract language is often vague and may generally reflect only a single perspective. For example, a contract may read as follows:

The hospital shall comply with the rules, policies, and procedures that the company has established or will establish, including but not limited to UR precertification of elective admissions and procedures, claims payment review, and hospital admissions as outlined in the hospital procedure manual (as modified from time to time).

The hospital agrees to participate in, as requested, and to abide by the company's UR, patient management, quality improvement programs, and all other related programs and decisions with respect to all members. Noncompliance with any of these requirements will relieve the payers and the members from any financial liability for all or any portion of the admission.

This terminology—which comes from excerpts of several contracts—is intended to put the hospital in a defensive posture, subject to the payer's whims. Every line in the plan's contract is designed to benefit the plan—not the hospital—so consider every provision to be negotiable and review each one carefully. UR terms are rarely addressed during negotiations, so although contract managers may walk out of negotiations feeling pleased that they agreed on the highest rates possible, the costs associated with complying with the UR requirements may not have been considered or discussed. The contracting team generally does not know what questions to ask, what terms to avoid, and what contingencies to cover. This lack of attention to the complexities of UR activities will come at great expense to the hospital.

The value of contract addendums

The provider manual stipulates the policies and procedures used to collect information about the full scope of the patient's episode of care, all the way from precertification to discharge. However, the same market power that the contract manager exercised in negotiating fair payment rates can be leveraged to modify the insurer's UR requirements. Hospitals can request contract addenda to make changes to these policies, and in the current economy, more hospitals are insisting on terms that are balanced and fair. Note, however, that it is not feasible to amend the provider manual, which is typically a generic document applicable to hospital markets across the country.

Contract negotiations can make or break a hospital, because in addition to setting the price list for services provided to the insurer's members, the negotiations also affect the resources that the provider expends to comply with the contract terms. These negotiations are critical in a competitive market, with significant implications for the organization, the patients, and the communities served. Facilities have been known to shut their doors because they passively negotiated and accepted whatever rates a payer offered. It's also been well publicized when negotiations result in a standoff and the hospital or payer walks away, leaving communities stranded. Hospital contract managers generally regard payers as being the hospital's bank— payers hold the money and control the processes.

When the contract manager goes into discussions with the payer, their priorities include setting a rate schedule that works for the hospital, crafting contract terms that simplify claims processing, and protecting against arbitrary denials. It is best to approach the process with a win-win attitude—there are plenty of opportunities to fashion contract provisions that benefit both the plan and the provider. Both parties should recognize that the contract must include terms that define the parties' mutual obligations for greater administrative efficiencies, such as the timeliness of payment and improvements in claims processing, and both are expected to walk out of the room having successfully negotiated a contract that allows each to profit. Hospital representatives also look for ways to improve contract language to cover payment for high-cost drugs, new technologies, sophisticated procedures, and medical devices. Note that, although the chief financial officer or contract manager gets knee-deep in financial discussions, it is rare that they discuss the peripheral issues of UR requirements.

No matter who negotiates these commercial insurer contracts for the hospital, they need to have sufficient data to support their position regarding addendum language and to maximize the UR team's results. The negotiator should use objective information on volumes, payer responsiveness, and denial history to support requests for language changes. For example, if there is little history of clinical denials for a particular payer, then language can be added to reduce the frequency of information requests. Figure 2.3 is a sample of provider-/payer-negotiated language that was used in past contract addendums that balances the payer's need for information and the provider's need for efficiency.

■ Figure 2.3

Sample of win-win utilization review language

It is agreed that should these utilization guidelines conflict with any other part of the agreement or amendments thereto, including but not limited to the INSURER'S provider manual, this policy statement shall prevail.

Authorization

Upon member admission, hospital shall provide notification to the payer electronically through the insurer's secure portal/email address to telephonically to the payer's designated representative. Within 24 hours of admission notification, hospital shall electronically forward clinical information supporting the patient's status as inpatient or outpatient. Payer shall issue an authorization decision within 8 hours confirming or denying admission status. Once confirmed, regardless of payer's subsequent determination, Payer shall be responsible for full payment of submitted claim.

Sample of win-win utilization review language (cont.)

Clinical review

{PAYER} may provide either on-site or electronic review of their inpatients. {PAYER} will accept electronic transmission of clinical reviews of their inpatients and will actively participate in discharge planning as requested by the {HOSPITAL}.

In the case of on-site clinical review, the {PAYER'S} reviewer shall meet with the patient's case manager or utilization reviewer to discuss findings at the conclusion of the review.

In the case of telephonic or electronic review under an MS-DRG, discounted FFS, or per diem contract, {HOSPITAL} will provide an initial clinical review within 24 hours or one business day of the notification of admission. Clinical information may be provided to {PAYER} using a secure electronic format or secure payer portal.

If an inpatient admission or continued stay is denied by the payer concurrently, the provider shall be given the opportunity to have a peer-to-peer discussion with the payer within 1 business day. This discussion may be conducted by any physician caring for the patient or any physician designated by the provider to represent them.

{PAYER} and {HOSPITAL} shall designate a primary contact person to provide and receive clinical information.

{HOSPITAL} and {PAYER} shall provide telephone numbers, email addresses, or other contact information for weekend and after-hours clinical reviews.

Initial and any concurrent reviews will be performed using current edition of InterQual® criteria. {HOSPITAL} acknowledges that out-of-state {PAYER} plans may use a different UR guideline or clinical criteria; however, {HOSPITAL} shall continue to provide information under InterQual guidelines.

Commercial criteria sets may not be modified by payer and as specified within the criteria, physician judgment may override them to approve inpatient admission.

{PAYER} may approve admission for selected diagnoses without requiring an initial clinical review.

Initial clinical reviews will contain the following information:

- Patient identification data
- Pertinent abnormal labs, vital signs, or imaging results used to define the InterQual criteria that the patient meets to qualify for inpatient admission or observation services
- Any IV fluids, medications, procedures, or treatments used to define the InterQual criteria the patient meets
- Preliminary discharge plan
- Medically necessary observation stays cannot exceed 48 hours.

For all inpatient services reimbursed by a DRG or Case Rate, a readmission to the same acute facility within three (3) days of the discharge from the first admission will be subject to clinical reviews if the readmission is determined to be for a related diagnosis or for a complication arising out of the first admission.

If a covered indivudal is readmitted furing the three (3) day postdischarge period, and the readmission stay is determined to have been preventable by provider actions that were not properly performed or omitted, then hospital shall only be reimbursed for the higher-weighted DRG admission. This readmission policy excludes the following: planned readmissions, patient transfers from one acute care hospital to another, patient discharged from the hospital against medical advice on the first admission, and cancer diagnoses. If the readmission is due to a failure of a contracted payer provider (SNF, HHA, DME) to provide services as required, the hospital will be held harmless and paid for both admissions in full.

Contracts and UR

For commercial payers, contractual arrangements generally dictate coverage and payment requirements. Employers will set general coverage and cost guidelines, which are then developed by the insurer and negotiated with the providers. As a result, one patient with insurance A may have different coverage, precertification requirements, and copayment than another patient who has insurance A but has a different plan type.

Because the typical hospital contract manager or health system contract coordinator has little knowledge of UR activities, someone with the requisite knowledge of the terms and provisions governing UR should be part of the negotiating team or, at a minimum, a member of the preparatory team. Because the UR language contained in the provider manual will affect the UR workflow and the extent of information demanded by the payer, we suggest that the lead UR specialist and department director meet with the contract manager prior to any negotiations to sensitize him or her to the implications of the provider manual directives. Be prepared to offer alternatives and to ask to be part of the nonfinancial negotiations. Consider the following categories of contract terms during preparatory strategy sessions:

1. Verification of eligibility: The contract should clarify how eligibility of coverage will be verified in a timely manner and should include the payer's responsibilities for payment when the provider has taken the necessary steps, but the payer is in error, or when services are provided in an emergency situation before eligibility can be verified.

   Example: The payer will be bound by its confirmation of eligibility as evidenced by the payer's identification card unless the provider has actual knowledge that the member is not eligible for covered services.

2. Medical necessity: Underlying most medical necessity determinations is the question of which standards will be used as a first-level review to determine whether an admission or continuing stay may be appropriate. To provide objective guidance, nationally recognized guidelines have been developed based on medical literature and professional practice guidelines. The most recognized and frequently used guidelines are Hearst's MCG Care Guidelines or Change Healthcare's Inter-Qual®, which have been validated by research and decades of clinical use. InterQual is a first-level screening tool that uses evidence-based, condition-specific criteria as well as the expected findings and interventions (formerly referred to as severity of illness; intensity of services). MCG defines optimal care guidelines based on evidence-based best practices for treating conditions that require the level of care being provided.

   The key here is to avoid allowing the payer to define medical necessity according to their own arbitrary cost criteria or allowing them to bypass secondary physician review. Both InterQual and MCG Care Guidelines are designed as screening criteria and specify that patients who do not pass the screening criteria should have a secondary review by a physician. This second step is often ignored, resulting in the payer's hasty determination of ineligibility for payment. Then all the back-end rework begins to appeal the payer's decision. Medical necessity provisions must be written to align the interests of the payer with those of the provider and the patient using evidence-based clinical content.

   Medical necessity based on information gathered at the time of admission is generally accepted as the basis for hospital level of care. However, there are some payers who deny payment based on final diagnosis rather than presenting diagnosis, as they will say that the principal diagnosis at discharge did not warrant hospital level of care. The Uniform Hospital Discharge Data Set clearly states that the principal diagnosis is the "condition established *after study* to be chiefly responsible for occasioning the admission of the patient to the hospital for care" (italics added).

   Example: The payer agrees that a request for specified acute care services made by a qualified practitioner who provides sufficient information consistent within generally acceptable professional medical standards and MCG Care Guidelines—and not primarily for the convenience of the patient, physician, or other healthcare providers—will not be subject to pre-authorization clinical review.

3. Transitions of care: Hospitals are often held financially responsible for the course of a patient's post-acute care with readmission penalties and denial of payment for the second admission. However, many payers limit resources available to patients for post-acute care, such as limiting SNF and home care agency choices or denying long-term acute care hospitalization admission. These limits leave the patient at high risk for readmission. Because the hospitalized patient doesn't relate directly with the payer, he or she may hold the hospital responsible for any benefit deficits. If the patient is a Medicare beneficiary, such an event will probably affect the hospital's patient satisfaction scores. The case management staff should review the network of preferred post-acute care providers for each payer along with any applicable criteria and provide feedback to the contracting staff if the list is not as comprehensive as their members may need it to be. Knowledge of post-acute disposition by payer is a valuable resource because it can provide objective information about where the payer's members went at discharge and whether there is a correlation between post-acute choices and readmissions. This is the value of having disposition codes by payer available during negotiations to objectively demonstrate need.

4. Payer delays: Another reported abuse of the payer's leverage is the delay by the payer in authorizing procedures, medications, or an approved post-acute plan. The provider cannot accept the patient until the payer provides the authorization number even when the post-acute provider is an approved member of the payer's network, and even when all the paperwork has been completed to the satisfaction of the post-acute provider and the hospital. Stalling tactics by the payer mean that the patient is warehoused in the hospital at the hospital's expense unless the contract language provides protection against the costs.

   Addenda example: Payer will coordinate the physician-ordered placement for SNFs, durable medical equipment, home health, rehab, or dialysis with their own vendors; issue timely and appropriate authorization to the vendors; and communicate the arrangement to the hospital via fax, predesignated telephone, or secure electronic transmission. Per diem reimbursement of $1,650 will be made for each day of delay that results in the payer's member needlessly remaining in the hospital.

5. Denial notifications: Following the lead of the RACs and the MACs, commercial insurers are increasingly auditing and denying hospital services, even after providing concurrent authorization for the services. UR specialists reading this book can likely attest to this fact of life when they are asked to investigate a denial for an admission and continuing stay that they had personally gotten approved. The payer may also claim that the clinical information contained in the medical record differs from the information provided at the time of the certification.

   Payers often review denial appeals internally—often using the same person who issued the denial in the first place. The payer's position on this issue restricts the opportunity for an objective assessment of medical necessity. Therefore, the contract should include terms and conditions for the hospital to appeal to an external review organization if the appeal is denied. Denial and appeal policies should be clearly delineated in the contract and reviewed by the personnel who will handle appeals at the hospital.

   It should also be noted that in the case of MA plans, the *Medicare Managed Care Manual,* Chapter 4, section 10.16 states that "if the plan approved the furnishing of a service through an advance determination of coverage, it may not deny coverage later on the basis of a lack of medical necessity." A recent trend has been seen where MA plans contract with external audit agencies to review paid claims, even those where authorization was provided. Unless these auditors find that the information provided to obtain the authorization was unsubstantiated, a denial cannot be issued and, if so, would violate Medicare regulations and could result in action by CMS against the MA plan (CMS, 2016).

6. Payment rates: Although payment rates are usually within the purview of the finance team, it is important to understand the interplay between status determinations and payment. For Medicare patients, the rules for status determination are based on one set of federal regulations. We also know that because the current Medicare payment system adds additional payments, such as medical education and disproportionate share, onto inpatient admissions but not outpatient services, the inpatient payment always exceeds the outpatient payment. But every commercial payer, as noted, can establish their own status rules, and varying provisions in a contract can result in varying patterns of reimbursement for the same service offered as inpatient or outpatient. If a particular payer contract pays inpatient services based on a per-admission basis but outpatient services are paid as a percent of charges, there is a high likelihood that the payment to the hospital for an outpatient surgery may exceed the inpatient payment. In that case, asking for prior authorization for inpatient admission makes no sense. The patient will receive the same care as inpatient or outpatient, so the higher reimbursement should be the goal.

Contract database

Once negotiations are completed, the contract manager should maintain a database of all contracts so they can easily access the contracting terms and key provisions applicable to UR activities (see Figure 2.4). This database should be regularly shared with the UR specialists, case managers, and the post-acute resource center personnel to streamline hospital-payer processes. The matrix includes highlights of the benefits, in-network providers, payment methodology, and contacts at that insurance company to efficiently provide UR and case management support to the patient and the physicians. Hospitals can often avoid delays in discharging patients—and avoid patient disappointment—by providing to patients who require post-acute care at a SNF, home care, or a transfer to a higher level of care information about the available choices for that care approved by their insurer.

■ Figure 2.4

	Original Contract Date/ Last Renewal Date	Is clinical required? Who to call?	Payer UR Contact	Inpatient Med/Surg	Outpatient Surgery	ICU/CCU Rates	OBS Covered?	Outpt Radiolo Rate?	Post Acute Benefits – Preferred Providers		
				Payment method	Payment method	Payment Method			HHC	SNF	Acute Rehab
Aetna US Healthcare	6/1/97 9/3/17	Clinical precert only for cardiac A.Smith 555-1212	Arlene G. 555-1212	DRG	Fee schedule	Carve out 20% discount with stop-loss >$50K	Yes - part B + obs hrs	Yes Separate contract	Yes-Devon Home Svcs	Yes – Lincoln Gdens	Yes w/ $500 ded
Aetna Mgd MediCAID	7/1/95 9/30/16	Clinical precert 48 hrs via ROCS B.Clark 555-1212	Robert G 555-1212	Per Diem	Fee schedule	Per Diem	Fixed fee	Schedule	Yes but only with Home-mark	Yes Limited	NO

	Original Contract Date/ Last Renewal Date	Is clinical required? Who to call?	Payer UR Contact	Inpatient Med/Surg	Outpatient Surgery	ICU/CCU Rates	OBS Covered?	Outpt Radiolo Rate?	Post Acute Benefits – Preferred Providers		
America's Health Plan	6-1-94 Continuing renewal w/90 day out notice	Clinical precert peds only S.Anthony 555-1212	Anthony D 555-1212	20% discount from charges	20% discount from charges	12.75 % discount from charges	Yes – bundled per diem	Yes	No	Yes	Y w/ $500 ded
BC BS Century Preferred	10/1/94 Continuing renewal w/90 day out notice	No precert required	Mr. P 555-1212	Per Diem	fee schedule	22% discount from charges	No – Part B only	Yes	Yes- Devon Home Svcs	Yes – Refer to Web site	Y – up to 30 days
BC BS ACO	11/17/16 ACO Shared Savings	Precert required + min of 48 hrs pre-elective procedure	Sarah Mellon – ACO TPA office 555-1212	FFS DRG Bonus benchmark PM/PM 2018 Risk share	FFS APC Bonus benchmark PM/PM 2018 Risk share	FFS DRG Bonus benchmark PM/PM 2018 Risk Share	Per diem. 2 MN max	Capitated	Contact ACO CM Liaison Shirley Adams prior to any referral		
BC Family Plan Managed MediCAID	9/1/01 Continuing renewal w/60 day out notice	Precert within 24 hrs	Barb Q 555-212	DRG	APC 2017	DRG	No – part B only	Schedule	No	No	No
BC Workers Comp PPO	9/1/01 9/1/17	Precert all with WC CaseMrg A.Green 555-1212	Will assign CM. Call Anne 555-1212	15% discount from charges	15% discount from charges	15% discount from charges	Yes	Capitated	Yes	Yes	Yes

Source: Reprinted with permission from Stefani Daniels, RN, MSNA, ACM, CMAC, founder and senior advisor at Phoenix Medical Management, Inc., in Pompano Beach, Florida.

Case management and UR staff should have access to this information so that if an issue arises with the payer relative to the revised contract language, it can be addressed immediately, and the payer can be held accountable to the terms of the contract. The database should also include calendar dates for expiration and renegotiation of each contract. If the contractual UR obligations need to be revisited, many contracts have provisions that automatically extend the contract ("evergreen contracts") unless notice of intent to renegotiate is provided in advance. Every director of case management, UR specialist, or revenue cycle chairperson should promote inclusion of a notice of intent to renegotiate in every commercial contract as part of the preparatory discussions with the contract manager.

These contract issues illustrate the crucial partnership that must develop between the UR staff and the revenue cycle team. The work of each closely interfaces with the duties of the other, and collaboration creates a win-win situation for both.

References

Centers for Medicare & Medicaid Services (CMS). (2014, May). Are you a hospital inpatient or outpatient? Retrieved from *https://www.medicare.gov/Pubs/pdf/11435.pdf*.

CMS. (2016). Chapter 4: Benefits and Beneficiary Protections. *Medicare Managed Care Manual.* Retrieved from *https://www.cms.gov/Regulations-and-Guidance/Guidance/Manuals/Downloads/mc86c04.pdf*.

CMS. (2018). CMS-3317-RCN. Medicare and Medicaid Programs; Revisions to Requirements for Discharge Planning for Hospitals, Critical Access Hospitals, and Home Health Agencies; Extension of Timeline for Publication of Final Rule. Retrieved from *https://public-inspection.federalregister.gov/2018-23922.pdf*.

CMS. (2019). CMS-3317-F and CMS-3295-F. Medicare and Medicaid Programs; Revisions to Requirements for Discharge Planning for Hospitals, Critical Access Hospitals, and Home Health Agencies, and Hospital and Critical Access Hospital Changes to Promote Innovation, Flexibility, and Improvement in Patient Care. Retrieved from *https://www.federalregister.gov/documents/2019/09/30/2019-20732/medicare-and-medicaid-programs-revisions-to-requirements-for-discharge-planning-for-hospitals*.

CMS. (2020). Fact sheet: Estimated improper payment rates for Centers for Medicare & Medicaid Services (CMS) programs. Retrieved from *https://www.cms.gov/newsroom/fact-sheets/2020-estimated-improper-payment-rates-centers-medicare-medicaid-services-cms-programs*.

CMS. (2021). Fast facts: Original Medicare persons served by type of service. Retrieved from *https://www.cms.gov/Research-Statistics-Data-and-Systems/Statistics-Trends-and-Reports/CMS-Fast-Facts*.

Freed, M., Damico, A., and Neuman, T. (2021). "A Dozen Facts About Medicare Advantage in 2020." Kaiser Family Foundation. Retrieved from *www.kff.org/medicare/issue-brief/a-dozen-facts-about-medicare-advantage-in-2020/*.

Hirsch, R. M. (2018, April 5). Hospital with 0.7% error rate hit with $1.88 million False Claim Act settlement. RAC Monitor. Retrieved from *https://www.racmonitor.com/hospital-with-0-7-error-rate-hit-with-1-88-million-false-claim-act-settlement*.

Office of Inspector General (OIG). (2015). OIG policy statement regarding hospitals that discount or waive. Retrieved from *https://oig.hhs.gov/compliance/alerts/guidance/policy-10302015.pdf*.

CHAPTER 3

The Business of Healthcare

Utilization Review and the Revenue Cycle

Mastery of the revenue cycle process is not a core job requirement for utilization review (UR) specialists, but understanding how hospitals and physicians get paid—as well as their patients' financial obligations—will allow the UR specialist to provide services that are more patient-centered and optimized for the organization. Although providing care to patients in a technologically advanced system is complex, this task can pale in comparison to the work the revenue cycle carried out to get payment for that care. Members of the revenue cycle face constant and complex challenges, from the initial encounter with the patient to obtain and verify their insurance coverage, to the preparation of a claim based on medical record documentation, to the end of the cycle, where staff collect and handle payment. And if the claim is rejected or denied after payment, a whole new set of challenges appear that again will require the joint efforts of the UR and finance teams.

Our nation's banking and financial system is well designed and interconnected with those of other countries, but our healthcare and health insurance systems are fragmented and disconnected. Each patient who walks into the hospital can have a different insurer that issues a different type of insurance identification card containing different amounts of information about that patient's coverage. It's possible to walk into a store in nearly any country in the world and use a credit card to pay for a purchase, and the merchant can get an immediate verification that payment will be forthcoming; however, no such system exists for health insurance in the United States.

Electronic health record (EHR) systems were supposed to help address this issue by being interconnected, but information in the EHR about a patient's care is rarely accessible to providers who are not affiliated with the hospital where that information was collected. One of this book's authors served as the EHR physician champion for his hospital and physician practice starting in the early 2000s, and at the time, vendors of both hospital and physician practice EHRs claimed that their products would be designed to the standards of Health Level Seven International, which would allow the systems to share health information seamlessly. Yet, to this day, that goal has not been met.

This lack of interoperability also applies to the healthcare payment system. There are myriad payment structures for healthcare, and those for the hospital rarely align with those for the physician. Patients are often unaware of what their health insurance covers and usually do not know which providers are contracted with their payer. It has literally taken an act of Congress to get insurers to ensure that their provider directories are accurate. The No Surprises Act passed in 2020 requires that insurers verify the listings in their directories at least once every 90 days. That confusion even extends to the pharmacy, where the same prescription can have a different out-of-pocket cost every time the patient refills it, sometimes leaving even the pharmacist unable to explain the patient obligation.

This chapter will provide an overview of revenue cycle issues that may interest the UR specialist. Do not consider this overview to be a definitive guide, however, as regulations change frequently and are subject to interpretation.

What is the revenue cycle?

According to the Healthcare Financial Management Association, the revenue cycle is defined as "all administrative and clinical functions that contribute to the capture, management, and collection of patient service revenue." The responsibilities of the revenue cycle team include the following:

- Determining patient identity and eligibility
- Obtaining accurate demographics
- Collecting patients' copays
- Certifying appropriateness for acute care
- Ensuring documentation specificity
- Coding claims correctly
- Tracking and monitoring claims
- Collecting payments
- Reporting denials
- Appealing denied claims

Google the term and you will see many images describing the dynamic revenue cycle process graphically. But it is rare to find any mention of UR in the mix.

Yet, there is an interdependent relationship between UR and revenue cycle. The UR process during the hospital stay is dependent on the revenue cycle team to ensure the patient's demographics and insurance information is accurate and confirmed so that authorization can be obtained if necessary and post-hospital transitions of care can be arranged within the patient's network. The revenue cycle depends on the UR process to ensure that payer authorization or notification is completed, if required, and often relies on the UR team to process denials and prepare appeals. And finally, the revenue cycle depends upon verification of medical necessity in order to complete its purpose: collection of full claim payment.

In the past, the activities associated with the revenue cycle remained hidden within the bowels of the hospital's business office, but as the demands from payers and regulators have increased, the people and processes associated with the revenue cycle have become more apparent. Given the responsibilities identified in the bulleted list at the beginning of this section, the connection between the UR team and the revenue cycle is increasingly evident in today's healthcare world. This is why we're seeing and support the shift of UR activities from its traditional position with case management to a position within finance/revenue cycle.

Revenue cycle team members

There is a distinction between the management of revenue cycle activities and the structure of a revenue cycle team. The value of consolidating revenue cycle–related activities under a vice president of revenue cycle is recognized as an industry standard and allows organizations of all types and sizes to streamline processes and optimize revenue. The structure and size of revenue cycle teams, on the other hand, depends upon the size of the organization. In larger hospitals or integrated delivery systems, there may be an enterprisewide revenue committee, which generally includes the chief financial officer (CFO), vice president of managed care contracting, director of access management, director of professional billing, director of patient financial services (PFS), and vice president of revenue cycle management. In small- to medium-sized hospitals, the typical revenue cycle team is led by a director of revenue cycle management and includes the director of PFS, director of access management, case management director (if the case management program structurally incorporates UR and clinical documentation integrity [CDI]), appeals coordinator, and various clinical department heads. In recent years, hospital financial teams have added dedicated revenue integrity teams whose duty it is to ensure that processes are in place to make certain the organization receives accurate and compliant reimbursement for every service, preventing revenue leakage, revenue degradation, and compliance risk.

A successful revenue cycle requires the participation of every hospital program and department that generates billable expenses and affects complete and accurate payment. If any player in the cycle fails to do his or her job correctly, that failure will affect the outcome of every subsequent player. Incorrect data entry (e.g., insurance information, patient demographics), incomplete documentation, coding errors, or simply a failure to understand how each person's job affects the revenue of the institution can result in rework, delays, and costly mistakes.

Revenue cycle, UR, and access management

A successful revenue cycle begins with a robust access management program. The admissions/registration team typically handles patient eligibility determinations, accurate capture of all demographics, and copay collection. The admissions/registration team is also integral to the UR process, because the UR process itself is often determined by the demographics collected and recorded in the registration process. If the information is not accurate or complete when it is collected initially, it will affect the rest of the process. Unfortunately, this problem is common. Based on the informal and unscientific surveys we've done at hospitals over the past 20 years, we estimate that 40% of face sheet information generated through the admissions office is incorrect. Most of the time, the UR specialist or case manager must stop what they are doing to correct the information, which unfortunately does not remedy the problem going forward. We recommend printing every example of incorrect demographic information on a regular basis and then sitting down with the director of admissions/registrations to review the work that had to be done to correct errors or complete missing information. Without that feedback, we have found that admission/registration leaders will report a high accuracy rate, because the UR specialists and case managers are correcting the data. Demographic inaccuracy is particularly problematic when it occurs in insurance information, patient's full name, or family contact information. Incorrect insurance information heavily affects the UR specialist's work because there is no way of knowing what the patient's insurer expects in terms of UR requirements. It also affects the work of case management as they plan transitions of care, which can lead to delays in discharge or transfer.

The UR process for a patient with original Medicare is generally quite different than that for a patient with Medicare Advantage (MA) or another commercial insurer. The regular Medicare UR process is typically quite stable, whereas every other insurer may have its own distinct process outlined in its provider manual. For example, regular Medicare patients must have medical necessity for hospital care documented in the medical record and reviewed by the UR staff, but payer notification isn't required. For MA plans, the notification requirements vary, with some requiring notification only for inpatient admission, some requiring notification for inpatient admission and outpatient (observation) stays of more than 24 hours, and some requiring notification for any hospital care.

Hospitals do not always do a good job of ensuring that every employee knows his or her role in the organization's revenue cycle. Even if a formal revenue cycle team does not exist in your hospital, every worker—especially the members of the UR/CDI team—should know the effect of his or her job on the revenue cycle. A consistent UR workflow is critical for a successful revenue cycle. Creating such a workflow means training everyone on the UR team on a standard workflow that includes all tasks necessary to confirm eligibility for admission and continuing stay. Too often, workflow depends on the individual's preferences and past experiences rather than on the program's goals and those of the hospital it represents. If steps are missed or tasks are forgotten, the revenue cycle may be compromised and reimbursement may be delayed.

How Hospitals Are Paid

To understand the basics of how hospitals are paid, first separate patients by payer. Even though the number of companies offering health insurance has been declining over the past several years due to industry consolidation, each insurer has myriad plans with varying payment structures customized for plan sponsors. These payers and payment structures can generally be divided into two groups: government and commercial. However, many traditional government plans have been outsourced to commercial payers.

The most important government plan is Medicare. However, when discussing payment, understand that information about payment for Medicare only applies to patients with regular Medicare—it does not apply to Medicare beneficiaries who choose to enroll in a MA plan in which their benefits are administered by a private insurance company. MA plans should always be treated as commercial plans for statistical purposes because they are governed by a contract between the provider and the insurer, not by government regulations—although many insurers have adopted some of Medicare's reimbursement models. All data related to regular Medicare must be separated from data on MA plans. We are still amazed to find CFOs who group both populations together.

Medicaid is also a government plan, but unlike in the case of Medicare, each state sets its own coverage and payment policies, which makes generalizations about payment impossible. In addition, many states have contracted with commercial payers to develop managed Medicaid plans. Similar to MA plans, managed Medicaid plans are not administered by CMS or the state—they are managed by commercial insurance companies that contract with government agencies.

Regular Medicare

Payment for care provided to regular Medicare patients is the easiest to understand because a single set of rules applies nationwide. As described earlier in this book, Medicare has Parts A, B, C, and D to cover the various benefits. Most hospitals in the country are paid under a prospective payment system (PPS), with a fixed amount for each service or set of services. Some hospitals are PPS-exempt and paid with a different payment structure; these include cancer hospitals, children's hospitals, religious nonmedical healthcare institutions, and critical access hospitals. This book will discuss only those payment principles that apply to PPS hospitals.

Medicare payment for inpatient admissions

Inpatient admissions are paid under the diagnosis-related group (DRG) system. Medicare uses the Medicare Severity DRG (MS-DRG) system, which is specific to the demographics of the Medicare-insured population, whereas many commercial insurers use the All Patient Refined DRG system, which better accounts for patients of all ages and adjusts into severity categories. The DRG payment system is designed to compensate the hospital for the average cost of caring for the average patient within the DRG based on the average resources used to treat such patients. Although the hospital will receive a single payment for the whole admission based on the DRG, the hospital must still submit an itemized claim to Medicare that includes all services provided. Medicare uses the information on these claims to set rates in future years and to make outlier payments, which will be discussed later in the chapter.

The DRG assigned to an episode of care for a patient is determined after discharge based on the principal diagnosis, any secondary diagnoses, and any procedures performed during the admission. The principal diagnosis is defined by the Uniform Hospital Discharge Data Set as "that condition established after study to be chiefly responsible for occasioning the admission of the patient to the hospital for care" (CMS, 2020). There are 767 MS-DRGs for 2021, with most diagnoses grouped into three DRGs, called triads, where the base DRG represents the patient with no comorbidities or complications, the next higher-weighted DRG represents the presence of one or more specified comorbidities and/or complications, and the third and highest-weighted DRG represents the presence of one or more specified major comorbidities and/or complications. Each year CMS reviews DRG data and determines if additional DRGs are needed, as they did in 2021 when a DRG specific to chimeric antigen receptor T-cell immunotherapy, a new treatment for cancer, was added, or if DRGs can be condensed. Hospital coders use a system called a grouper to input all the diagnosis codes and procedure codes, and the grouper will look at the combination of codes and assign the appropriate DRG.

Calculating the payment to the hospital for the inpatient admission starts with the DRG. Each DRG is assigned a relative weight, which is then used to calculate a base payment rate. That base rate, which is based on the costs necessary for treating the average patient in that DRG in the previous year, is then adjusted by several variables, such as labor-related costs for the hospital's locality and, in some circumstances, cost of living. Hospitals that serve a large number of low-income patients will receive additional payment from the disproportionate share hospital (DSH) program. Hospitals that are approved as teaching hospitals receive an indirect medical education payment added on to each admission. If the hospital provides uncompensated care, there may be an additional payment provided.

There are also additional payments made or payments deducted from the DRG based on the Medicare programs that aim to move payment from a quantity-based system to a quality-based system. These programs include the Hospital Value-Based Purchasing Program, the Hospital Readmissions Reduction Program (HRRP), and the Hospital-Acquired Condition Reduction Program. There are additional payments for capital costs, including depreciation, interest, rent, and property-related insurance and taxes.

There are also additional payments made for new technology. Medicare approves a list of new technologies each year, and this list can include new medications, new procedures, or new devices whose costs have not yet been considered in the DRG weighting. If an approved new technology is used, an additional payment is made that is equal to 65% of the cost of the new technology, except for new antibiotics, which are paid at 75% of the cost. New technology payments generally are approved for three years, after which time CMS has accumulated enough data from claims and cost reporting to adjust DRG payments to account for these new technologies. CMS will also reassign DRGs as warranted to ensure reimbursement is adequate when the new technology payment sunsets, as has been done in the past with new cardiovascular device use.

Finally, certain PPS hospitals, designated as sole community providers, Medicare-dependent, low-volume, and rural referral centers receive additional payments to cover their added costs of operation in areas where they could not otherwise be financially viable and would leave communities without adequate healthcare.

Outlier payments

An outlier payment structure was developed to account for the difference between the average cost of caring for a patient and the patients who exceed that average cost by a large amount. If the cost of caring for a single patient exceeds a threshold amount set each year, then the hospital will receive an additional payment for that admission. That additional payment is generally 80% of the added costs over the threshold amount, so although the hospital does receive additional payment, the payment still amounts to less than the actual cost of providing that care. Commercial payers may also offer outlier payments if such payments are included in the contract.

There is a similar outlier payment system for outpatient services, but in that case the outlier payment is 50% of the amount that the costs exceed that threshold. Most of these cases will be high-cost, short-stay surgeries that are not eligible for inpatient admission.

The three-day payment window

An inpatient admission begins with the start of inpatient care pursuant to an inpatient order from a qualified practitioner. At face value, that would suggest that any services provided before the inpatient admission should be considered an outpatient service and would therefore be paid separately. Although those services are outpatient services, they do not generate any additional payment because of the three-day payment window, which states that "a hospital (or an entity that is wholly owned or wholly operated by the hospital) must include on the claim for a beneficiary's inpatient stay, the diagnoses, procedures, and charges for all outpatient diagnostic services and admission-related outpatient non-diagnostic services that are furnished to the beneficiary during the three-day (or one-day) payment window" (CMS, 6 May 2014). There is a one-day payment window for non-short-term acute care hospitals, but there is no payment window for critical access hospitals (CAH). For CAHs, all services prior to the inpatient admission are billed on an outpatient claim. This is an important distinction for CAHs, since their patients will be not only responsible for the Part A deductible for the inpatient admission but also for the 20% coinsurance for the outpatient services that were provided prior to the admission order.

There are some nuances to this rule. First, it specifically refers to entities owned or wholly operated by a hospital. Thus, the rule does not apply to entities that are owned by a health system, even if the health system owns both the entity and the hospital (unless the hospital itself operates the entity). Second, as the number of physician practices owned by hospitals increase, the facility fee charged when a patient visits a physician in the payment window may be subject to this rule (CMS, 14 June 2014). This would mean that if a patient who is scheduled for inpatient colon surgery on a Friday undergoes an imaging study on Wednesday, then the charge for the imaging would be placed on the inpatient claim even if the imaging study was unrelated to the surgery. On the other hand, if the patient was seen on Wednesday by their ophthalmologist whose practice was owned by the hospital for a scheduled check of their glaucoma, which is unrelated to the reason for admission, the facility fees associated with that visit would not be subject to the three-day rule.

Note that this rule specifies three calendar days, not 72 hours. If the admission occurs on Friday, services provided on Tuesday, Wednesday, and Thursday, regardless of their time, are subject to this rule. Also, note that although payment for services provided in the three-day window are bundled into the DRG payment, the inpatient admission begins on the date that inpatient care begins. These three days are also different from the three-day stay skilled nursing facility (SNF) requirement, as the days prior to admission cannot be counted as inpatient days when determining qualification for coverage of a Part A stay at a SNF.

Although there is a payment window that precedes inpatient admissions, there is no payment window following an inpatient discharge. Thus, any services provided to the patient after formal discharge from the hospital can be billed separately, even if they are provided on the day of discharge. These services cannot be related to the reason for the inpatient admission and delayed until after discharge in order to circumvent the payment system. For example, if a patient is hospitalized as inpatient for pneumonia and needs a CT scan of the chest for follow-up of their infection, the patient cannot be discharged and then proceed to the radiology department to complete the scan as an outpatient. On the other hand, if the patient was found to have an incidental thyroid nodule during their admission, they could be discharged, proceed to radiology for an ultrasound, and have that scan billed as an outpatient service. Because these situations are difficult for the billing and coding staff to differentiate, try not to provide outpatient services on the day of discharge unless the circumstances are compelling, and then only with clear communication with the billing staff.

Readmissions

CMS began penalizing hospitals for readmissions in 2012. Since that time, hospitals have worked extensively to reduce readmissions (CMS, 30 November 2017). Many believe that the HRRP is designed such that CMS would not pay for a readmission if a regular Medicare beneficiary is readmitted to a hospital within 30 days, but this is not entirely true. Instead, the HRRP weighs the hospital's expected readmission rate of inpatients admitted during a respective year against the hospital's observed or actual readmission rate. CMS then uses this information to calculate the hospital's readmission penalty and reduces payment for each admission to the hospital for three years. This means the hospital is paid the full DRG payment for the readmission up front but uses that readmission and other readmissions to calculate the potential penalty that will be assessed in future years.

According to Kaiser Health News, under HRRP, Medicare penalized half of United States hospitals for too many readmissions between the years 2016 and 2019. Retroactive to 1 October 2020, Medicare lowered a year's worth of payments to 2,545 hospitals. The average reduction is 0.69%, with 613 hospitals receiving a penalty of 1% or more (Rau, 2020).

In some instances, hospitals might lose revenue because the readmission penalty is based on the observed readmission rate compared to the expected readmission rate. Hospitals might also notice a reduction in DRG payments for 30-day readmissions. Hospitals that have implemented and invested money in readmission reduction initiatives might find that the cost of such initiatives outweighs the readmission penalty, resulting not only in lost revenue due to penalties but also in increased spending. Financial considerations aside, reducing preventable readmissions is the right thing to do. It should also be noted that if a patient who was an inpatient at one hospital gets admitted to another hospital within 30 days of discharge, the readmission will go into the first hospital's calculation of their readmission rate although they do not financially benefit from payment for the readmission.

Readmissions are not billed as new admissions if the patient is readmitted to the same hospital on the same calendar day as their discharge to be treated for symptoms related to or for evaluation and management of the prior stay's medical condition. In these instances, CMS instructs the hospital to combine the two admissions into one as if the patient were never discharged (CMS, 5 April 2013). If the patient returns to the hospital after the initial admission but presents with a problem unrelated to that admission, the second admission would not be rolled into the initial stay and should therefore be billed as a new admission with the applicable condition code.

Non-Medicare payers have a myriad of rules applicable to readmissions, which should be addressed in the payer contract, provider manual, or an addendum to the contract. Some payers will combine any readmission within a prespecified time period with the index admission, while some will pay the first admission but not the second. In other cases, the payer will review the readmission to determine if the readmission was related to the index admission and if the readmission was preventable and then decide if it should be paid. Others will consider a readmission to a hospital in the same health system as a readmission to the "same" hospital and deny payment for the second admission. This once again falls to your contracting team to ensure that the rules on payment for readmissions are fair and equitable.

The review of readmissions is often the work of specific teams within the hospital, but the UR team and case managers should take an interest in this. The cause of readmissions can be myriad, but, in general, it is important to find those readmissions where the hospital or medical team's actions contributed. Some of the most common patients to experience readmissions are those with heart failure (HF) or chronic obstructive lung disease (COPD). However, these patients' higher likelihood of readmission is understandable because, unlike patients with pneumonia or heart attack, COPD and HF are chronic conditions. COPD and HF patients are typically hospitalized due to exacerbation of their chronic disease and discharged when that has been stabilized. A patient such as this returning in 28 days would be much more likely due to another spontaneous exacerbation than anything that happened during their previous admission that should result in a penalty for the hospital. On the other hand, the HF patient who returns a week later with hypotension whose medication reconciliation reveals they were sent home on two angiotensin-blocking blood pressure medications was clearly due to a breakdown in process.

Readmissions and SDoH

It has also been suggested that readmissions are often the result of issues related to social determinants of health (SDoH). Inadequate insurance coverage, food insecurity, housing instability, language barriers, health literacy, discomfort with discharge, disabilities, and lack of social supports all contribute to an unplanned readmission as well as super-utilization of the emergency department (ED). Several recent studies show a positive correlation between SDoH and ED super-utilization and emphasize the importance of adopting the use of valid risk assessment tools to predict readmissions (Yongkang, 2020; Bensken, 2021).

Note that the 21st Century Cures Act gives CMS authority to change the HRRP to account for patient social risk, but it remains unclear whether the agency will move forward with doing so. CMS is currently studying the effect of individuals' social risk factors on value-based payment programs, although no time frame has been cited for reporting on their findings.

Although the SDoH may be coded with ICD-10-CM codes (all within the Z55–Z65 range), they do not currently affect DRG assignment. In the 2019 IPPS proposed rule, CMS proposed adding ICD-10-CM code Z59.0 (homelessness) as a comorbidity that would result in a change in DRG and additional payment to the hospital. Unfortunately, the proposal was not finalized. Even without this official designation as a "payable" comorbidity, it is important that this diagnosis, and all social determinants that influence a patient's health status, gets documented. Most importantly, coders must be reminded to add the code to the claim. Claim form information is the basis of most statistical data collected internationally. Therefore, only if all coders ensure that SDoH are appropriately coded will researchers be able to see the influences that the SDoH have on length of stay, cost of care, challenges in discharge, and so on. It is doubly important for local hospitals to have this information to evaluate and develop strategies to address the broader SDoH in the communities they serve. In fact, the importance of this information is demonstrated by the fact that the official coding guidelines allow the ICD-10-CM code for any SDoH to be placed on a claim based on documentation from any member of the care team, and not simply physicians, as is the case with medical diagnoses (AHA, 2019).

The UR team may also at times be involved in notifications to the payers of admissions and continuing stays. This can include arrangements for post-acute care. This also plays a role in readmissions if the home care company that is contracted with the payer does not show up for visits or the contracted skilled nursing facility is unable to handle the medical needs of the patient. In these situations, the hospital should not be held responsible for activities over which they have no control.

Post-Acute Care Transfer Payments (PACT)

Discharges are paid as transfers when the patient is transferred from acute to post-acute care at a skilled nursing facility, starts a home healthcare episode of care within three days, or is discharged to another inpatient setting. In these instances, the acute care hospital may not be paid the DRG rate. Rather, the hospital is paid twice the per diem rate for the first day of the hospital stay, and then it is paid the per diem rate for each subsequent day up to the total DRG amount.

The geometric mean length of stay (GMLOS) assigned to the patient's discharge DRG at the acute care facility provides a target transfer date. CMS' post-acute transfer (PACT) policy (formerly known as transfer DRGs) reduces inpatient payment if patients assigned to any of 280 qualifying DRGs are transferred to a post-acute care setting more than one day before the transfer date determined by the GMLOS and DRG. In those cases, the discharge DRG payment is divided by the GMLOS, and the resulting calculation is rounded to the nearest whole number to arrive at a per diem rate.

If an inpatient is transferred from an acute care hospital to be admitted as an inpatient at an accepting hospital, then the transferring hospital is paid based on the transfer payments outlined above. The accepting hospital is paid the full DRG payment unless the patient is later transferred to a SNF or starts a home health episode of care. In this case, the DRG payment to the accepting hospital will be subject to the post-acute transfer adjustment based on the length of stay at the accepting hospital.

Transfer payments are applied when the claim from the hospital includes a patient discharge status code, or discharge disposition codes, that invokes one of the aforementioned adjustments. These patient discharge status codes are applied to the claim based on the information in the medical record that is available to the coders. The accuracy of the codes becomes quite important from a revenue perspective: Most of the time, the coders will rely on the disposition code previously entered into the record at the time of discharge, usually by the discharging nurse.

Discrepancies often come to light when comparing anecdotal information about the extent of post-acute transfer logistics to an electronic report of the actual destinations. Inevitably, the percent discharged home without services belies the anecdotal reports—in fact, investigation generally uncovers widespread disregard for the accuracy of the patient discharge status codes. This disregard causes multiple problems: Not only does the data not correlate with the clinical staff's reports, but it also puts the hospital at compliance risk.

The discharge destination may also change postdischarge. For example, as we described before, if a patient is discharged with arrangements for home care services and then refuses to allow the home care staff into their home, no home health claim will be submitted and no post-acute transfer adjustment should be made. Hospitals should have processes in place to ensure that post-acute services listed on the claims were actually provided to the patient. If the services on the claim were not provided, then the claim can be adjusted, resulting in reversal of the reduction to the DRG payment. On the other hand, a patient may be discharged home with no home care but then contact their primary care physician who orders home care. If that home care episode of care begins within three calendar days of discharge, it is the hospital's responsibility to ascertain that and adjust its claim to indicate the correct patient discharge status code.

Accuracy and capture of patient discharge status codes are frequent issues in hospitals: Who is assigned responsibility for an accurate code? The patient's nurse? The case manager? The UR specialist? The unit clerk? The coder? There is no standard, but, based on our experience, responsibility is not routinely assigned. If we were asked to suggest the responsible party, it would be the discharging nurse, who, more than anyone else on the patient's care team, knows exactly where the patient is going at discharge. Then, as described previously, there must be a process to determine if there was any change after the patient left the hospital. The bottom line is that an accurate code affects payment, and Medicare Administrative Contractor edits could reveal patterns of incorrect codes and trigger an Office of Inspector General audit. We urge you to give close attention to the patient discharge status codes at your organization.

Round trip transfers or services "under arrangement"
Patients are often transferred to other hospitals for a higher level of care than can be provided at the hospital. As noted earlier, in many of these round-trip transfer cases there is a transfer agreement in place and the patient is transferred back to the originating facility after the specialized care is provided. For Medicare patients, this is not considered a transfer. This patient remains an inpatient at the originating facility, and the accepting hospital provides the necessary services "under arrangement." Those services are then placed on the originating facility's claim with the appropriate coding.

Patient financial liability for inpatient care
When considering the patient's financial obligation for their care, remember that many patients have a supplemental plan, either purchased separately, provided by their employer, or as a retirement benefit. There are currently 10 approved types of "Medigap" plans, with varying coverages and out-of-pocket liabilities,

making it almost impossible to calculate an individual's potential financial liability. The copayments and deductibles described here represent those for the patient who has no supplemental plan.

CMS determines patient liability for inpatient admissions annually using a deductible set for each episode of illness. An episode of illness starts on the day of inpatient admission and continues 60 days from the date of discharge from an inpatient hospital or a Part A SNF stay. That deductible is then due again if the patient starts another episode of illness. However, if the patient is readmitted 59 days after discharge, the original episode of illness continues, and the patient will not incur a new deductible.

For 2021, the inpatient deductible is $1,484. There is no coinsurance for the first 60 days of inpatient hospital care, but the next 30 days require a $371 coinsurance charge per day. At day 91, the patient may elect to start using their 60 lifetime reserve days, in which case they would also owe a $742 daily coinsurance, or they may assume the full financial responsibility for continued inpatient care.

The issue of patient financial liability is often raised in the emergency department when a patient is informed that they will be hospitalized. Depending on their source of information, they may have received incorrect information on the costs they may incur. In no circumstance should the admission decision be based on the patient's potential financial liability but solely on the regulations for status determinations provided by CMS or their payer.

Outpatient services

Just as the DRG system was developed for payment of inpatient services under the prospective payment system, payment for outpatient services has its own prospective payment system called the ambulatory payment classification (APC). As with the DRG system, CMS groups services with similar costs and characteristics into APCs. For example, a chest X-ray is in the same APC as an X-ray of the lumbar spine, as these X-rays have similar costs. The base payment for each APC can be found on Addendum B of the Outpatient Prospective Payment System (OPPS). As with DRGs, there is a formula for high-cost outpatient encounters to determine whether an outlier payment should be made in addition to the APC payment.

There is also a complex set of rules that can result in APCs being combined or packaged into other APCs. For example, if a patient is seen in the emergency department and has laboratory tests performed, each laboratory test is assigned to an APC, but the costs for the laboratory tests are packaged into a composite APC payment for the emergency department visit instead of being paid separately. If the patient came to the laboratory from their physician's office with an order for the same laboratory tests, the hospital would be paid for each test because there was no accompanying emergency department visit.

CMS assigns a status indicator to each outpatient Healthcare Common Procedure Coding System (HCPCS) code that identifies whether the services described are paid under the OPPS and, if so, whether payment is packaged or made separately. Status indicators can be accessed at *www.cms.gov/Medicare/Medicare-Fee-for-Service-Payment/HospitalOutpatientPPS/Addendum-A-and-Addendum-B-Updates.html.*

Comprehensive ambulatory payment classification

In 2015, CMS took packaging a step further and introduced the comprehensive APC (C-APC) payment structure. When CMS introduced the concept of C-APCs in the 2014 OPPS proposed rule, they stated the following:

> Beneficiaries think of a single service such as "getting my gall bladder removed" or "getting a pacemaker." We believe that defining certain services within the OPPS in terms of a single comprehensive service delivered to the beneficiary improves transparency for the beneficiary, for physicians, and for hospitals by creating a common reference point with a similar meaning for all three groups and using the comprehensive service concept that already identifies these same services when they are performed in an inpatient environment. (CMS, 2013, July 19)

Thus, for outpatient services that fall into a C-APC, the hospital will receive a single payment that will encompass all of the services that the patient receives from the beginning of care until discharge. CMS assigned many common outpatient surgeries (such as the gall bladder removal or pacemaker procedures mentioned in the proposed rule) to C-APCs. The specific rules governing C-APCs are beyond the scope of this book, but note that because a single payment encompasses all services provided to the patient during their stay, the UR specialist should ensure that the services provided are related to the primary reason for the patient's hospital visit and are not being done for convenience (that is, on a "while they are here" basis). For example, if a patient has an outpatient laparoscopic hysterectomy, which is assigned to C-APC 5361, and the physician orders a CT scan of the sinuses because the patient is already at the hospital, there will be no additional payment within that C-APC for the CT scan.

CMS also established a C-APC for patients who are hospitalized as outpatient with observation services, C-APC 8011. Most UR specialists will encounter this C-APC frequently. An outpatient must meet certain conditions for classification into this C-APC, including:

- They are referred for observation services from the emergency department or from a community physician
- They receive eight or more hours of observation services, exclusive of time spent receiving services whose description includes active monitoring
- The patient does not undergo a procedure that is assigned a status indicator of T or J1

As with other C-APCs, payment will include all services provided to the patient from their time of arrival at the hospital until discharge. For 2021, the base payment for C-APC 8011 (observation services) is approximately $2,283. In 2018, when the previous edition of this book was published, it was paid at $2,350. This decline in payment illustrates the way CMS calculates payments. The 2018 rate was based on claims data from 2016 and the 2021 rate from claims data in 2019. Between 2016 and 2019, hospitals around the country expended great effort to reduce the length of stay and unnecessary testing for patients receiving observation services. In turn, this lowered hospitals' costs of providing observation services. Therefore, based on claims data that reflected a lower average charge for observation stays, CMS adjusted reimbursement accordingly.

C-APCs and status indicators

If the patient undergoes a status indicator J1 procedure, such as a surgery, the payment for the surgery cancels out any payment for observation. For example, if a patient presents to the emergency department with abdominal pain and is treated as an outpatient with observation while undergoing evaluation but then undergoes a laparoscopic cholecystectomy and is discharged the next day, the payment for the encounter will be the same as it would be if the patient had presented electively for a laparoscopic cholecystectomy; according to the status indicator, the payment for the surgery, C-APC 5361, cancels out any payment for the observation care, C-APC 8011, as noted above.

There are also procedures assigned to status indicator T; in general, these procedures are paid separately unless performed during the same encounter as a J1 procedure. But CMS also set a rule that the performance of a T procedure precludes payment of C-APC 8011. For example, a patient presents with rectal bleeding, is placed as a hospital outpatient with observation services, and undergoes a status indicator T procedure, such as a colonoscopy. If the patient is discharged prior to the second midnight, then the T procedure precludes payment for the observation C-APC. In that case, the hospital will be paid for the emergency department visit, the colonoscopy, and any other services that are not bundled but will receive no payment for the observation services.

As with DRGs, adjustments made to APC payments are based on the hospital's labor costs, but unlike with DRGs, there are no added payments for items such as medical education or uncompensated care. There are also no penalties incurred for failing to meet any quality measures. This lack of added payment for education and uncompensated care is especially pertinent when a surgery is removed from the inpatient-only list. When a surgery that was inpatient-only is performed as outpatient, the reimbursement drops substantially. For example, when total knee arthroplasty (TKA) was removed from the inpatient-only list in 2018, a teaching hospital that was paid $25,000 for an inpatient TKA could see the reimbursement drop to $12,000 for the same surgery done as outpatient. The yearly changes to the inpatient-only list usually produce a myriad of these stark changes in reimbursement, leading to significant angst in the finance departments of hospitals around the country.

Claim Preparation

Hospitals and facilities, such as laboratories, home care agencies, durable medical equipment providers, etc., complete and submit a form called a UB-04, either electronically or on paper, to bill for services. This form includes most of the information that the payer needs to determine whether the service is covered, determine whether any special circumstances need to be considered, and pay the claim.

The UB-04 contains fields for diagnosis codes, procedure codes, the date the service was performed, and the charge for the service, along with the demographic information about the patient and the identity of the ordering providers. For hospital claims, the UB-04 has fields to indicate the date(s) of the beginning and end of the services provided to the patient. There is also a field for the date and time of inpatient admission and a space to indicate when a patient who is initially treated as outpatient with observation services is then admitted as an inpatient on a different day. For example, say that a patient who presents to the emergency department on September 2 at 4 p.m. begins observation services at 8 p.m. On the next day (September 3) at 2 p.m., it is determined that the patient requires continuing hospital care, and an admission order is written. The patient remains in the hospital as an inpatient until September 4 and is discharged home. In this case, form locator field 6 will indicate that the claim statement covers care from September 2 to September 4, and form locator fields 12 and 13 will indicate that the inpatient admission began on September

3 at 2 p.m. Occurrence span code 72 will also be added to indicate that the patient's hospital stay met the 2-midnight benchmark.

The UB-04 also contains fields for condition codes. There is a long list of such codes for many situations, from codes that indicate denial of an admission by the Quality Improvement Organization to those that indicate whether the patient is using their lifetime reserve days. All UR specialists are familiar with the condition code 44 (CC44) process to change an inpatient to outpatient as described in Chapter 2. While we often refer to condition code as a process, it is in fact simply a code that gets added to a claim to indicate to the payer that the patient's inpatient status was changed to outpatient after utilization review. Condition code W2 should be included on inpatient and outpatient Part B claims that are submitted after an inpatient admission is self-denied.

The UB-04 also includes fields for occurrence codes and occurrence span codes. Occurrence codes are rarely used, but they denote inpatient hospital days that are not medically necessary or are days spent waiting for a SNF bed to become available. Occurrence code M1 is placed on an inpatient claim that is self-denied. There are also fields for value codes and revenue codes, the purpose of which falls outside the scope of a UR specialist's needs.

Outpatient claim modifiers can be appended to a HCPCS or CPT code and may be placed on the claim to indicate that a service has been altered but that the HCPCS or CPT code still applies. For example, if an outpatient surgery is started but then terminated prior to completion, modifier 74 (discontinued outpatient hospital/ambulatory surgery center procedure after administration of anesthesia) is used.

Condition Code 44 vs. W2

Chapter 2 provided an overview of CC44, but claim preparation for these two circumstances warrants mention, as the UR team is involved in the process. For traditional Medicare, if a patient's status is changed during the hospital stay from inpatient to outpatient using the CC44 process established by CMS in 2004, the complete claim is billed as an inpatient stay. If the patient received any observation services via an order during the encounter, those hours would be included on the claim. The change from inpatient to outpatient, although changing the whole claim, does not change the inpatient hours to billable observation hours. If the patient received observation services prior to the inpatient admission order and then the status was changed back to outpatient, the observation hours prior to the admission order can be billed along with any observation hours that the patient may have received after the switch back to outpatient.

In the case of an inpatient admission that was determined after discharge to have been in the incorrect status through the formal UR process spelled out in 42 *CFR* 482.30(d), the claim preparation and submission requires three steps. Initially the claim must be prepared as an inpatient claim and submitted as a provider-liable claim with occurrence span code M1. Then two Part B claims are prepared, an outpatient Part B claim for all services prior to the inpatient admission order and an inpatient Part B claim for services after the admission order. The inpatient Part B claim must be billed with condition code W2, indicating to CMS that there are no pending appeals of the previously submitted inpatient claim. Once again, the only observation hours that should be on these claims are for observation services provided to the patient when their status was outpatient and there was an order for observation services. The hours the patient spent in the hospital after the inpatient admission order cannot be rebilled as observation hours.

Bundled Payment and Shared Savings Programs

In 2013, CMS rolled out the Bundled Payments for Care Improvement (BPCI) initiative to test innovative ways of paying for medical care (CMS, 6 December 2017). There were four models released, with each one covering a different type of episode of care in either a prospective or a retrospective payment arrangement. For example, Model 2 starts with an inpatient admission and covers all inpatient and outpatient services provided to the patient from the date of admission until the 90th day after discharge. Payment for this model occurs via a retrospective payment bundle. In contrast, Model 4 is a prospective payment for an inpatient admission that covers all services furnished by the hospital, physician, and other practitioners during that episode of care. The BPCI program is unique in that it allows providers to share in the financial savings that were the result of their care coordination efforts without the risk of violating anti-kickback laws. All BPCI programs are voluntary, and each group is able to choose which patient categories would be part of the program.

In 2018, CMS initiated the BPCI Advanced program, which will include 32 inpatient and outpatient clinical episodes. As with BPCI, all costs incurred within the 90-day period after the episode begins will be compared to a target cost, with reconciliation resulting in either a positive amount—which will be paid to the convener (either a hospital or a physician group)—or a negative amount, which must be paid back to CMS. As with BPCI, CMS will monitor quality standards that must be met in order for hospitals or physician groups to receive an incentive payment. The UR staff may find that physicians become more interested in advancing patients through the continuum of care and more conscious of the use of post-acute resources for patients in these clinical episodes.

In 2015, CMS created a mandatory payment program called the Comprehensive Care for Joint Replacement (CJR) program (CMS, 22 December 2017). This program was initiated in 67 metropolitan service areas, and any patient at hospitals in the specified areas who had a qualifying joint replacement surgery that fell into DRG 469 or 470 was considered to be part of the program. CJR looked at total costs incurred from the date of the surgery until 90 days after discharge, including all spending on physician services during the hospital stay and after discharge, the inpatient hospitalization, and all post-acute care. The total spending was then compared to the historic costs for these patients from the hospital and the nation, and any savings above a threshold amount were returned to the hospital to share with collaborators. If the costs exceeded the threshold in years two and beyond, the hospital and collaborators would have to pay back a portion of the excess costs.

In order to ensure that these models do not compromise patient care, patients must be given notification that they are "participants" in a Medicare innovation program and that quality measures are being monitored. As an added benefit, CMS waived the three-day stay requirement for access to a SNF for post-hospital rehabilitation in the second year of the CJR or BPCI program if the patient chooses a SNF with a rating of three stars or more.

In 2016, CMS finalized a plan to expand the mandatory bundled payment programs to include admissions for acute myocardial infarction, hip fractures, and coronary artery bypass surgery (CMS, 19 May 2017). However, in December 2017, CMS officially cancelled this expansion, along with trimming the CJR program in half, which suggests a shift away from mandatory programs and toward voluntary programs when testing innovative payment methods.

In the intervening years, CMS has modified many of the bundled payment programs. For example, in 2021, CMS removed the volunteer participation from CJR and limited it to mandatory participants. They also added outpatient total joint arthroplasty surgery as part of the program, including allowing these outpatients to have access to Part A SNF benefits for rehabilitation if needed (CMS, 2021).

In 2017, CMS started adjusting payments in the HRRP to account for a hospital's percentage of patients who are dual eligible (which means that they are insured by both Medicare and Medicaid). This change is the first recognition by CMS that SDoH significantly affect patient health and is a first step toward having adjustments applied to bundled payment programs that calculate performance rates based on the comparison of expected to observed outcomes. SDoH are factors that influence health but are not medical, such as homelessness, illiteracy, death of a family member, divorce, and history of abuse. Unlike medical diagnoses, documentation from any clinician, including case managers and UR specialists, can be used to support codes for SDoH. Inclusion of all social determinants will ensure that a hospital's data accurately represents its patients' demographics.

Accountable Care Organizations (ACO)

An ACO is a voluntary program where providers can share in the savings if they are able to reduce costs of care for a panel of patients throughout the year. CMS uses historical data to set a benchmark spending amount, and any amount that falls below that benchmark represents savings. There are various models of ACOs, as some allow shared savings without responsibility for losses (upside gain only), and some allow increased shared savings when providers take on partial responsibility for costs if they exceed the benchmark (upside gain and downside risk). As with the other bundled payment programs, CMS monitors quality and allows patients to choose their own provider to ensure that patient care is not compromised. These programs are evolving on a yearly basis as The Center for Medicare & Medicaid Innovation (CMMI) reviews results from ongoing programs and monitors programs developed and tested in the private sector. The CMMI webpage allows one to see the various programs and apply to participate *(https://innovation.cms. gov/innovation-models/aco)*.

Telehealth

Until recently, the use of telehealth—the provision of medical care remotely using audio and/or visual devices—was limited. Most payers, including Medicare, limited telehealth use to rural areas where patients were unable to access needed specialty care in their community or nearby cities. Billing rules were stringent, requiring the patient to reside in a rural area and go to an "originating site," such as a physician office or hospital clinic, and communicate from there with a physician at a "distant site," such as the physician's office or a hospital clinic. The originating site would be paid a nominal fee for hosting the patient and providing the secure connection, and the physician would bill for their professional fee.

The COVID-19 public health emergency led to a marked relaxation of the rules, allowing expanded access to telehealth. CMS and payers allowed any type of visit to be performed with telehealth, removing the originating site requirements and permitting physicians to perform the visit from any location. The Office of Civil Rights also issued temporary enforcement discretion on the use of non-HIPAA-certified means of communication, allowing visits to be performed with applications available on smartphones and computers. In addition, billing rules were modified to allow coding of a telehealth visit as if the patient was seen in person.

The future of telehealth after the public health emergency is unclear. CMS has broad discretion to waive federal regulations during a public health emergency, but once that emergency expires, all prior rules and regulations resume. CMS will then have to decide which rules should be permanently changed and proceed through the normal rule-making process. Many are advocating for making the temporary telehealth changes permanent, but others caution that widespread long-term use of telehealth without any data on the patient outcomes is premature. Reimbursement for telehealth services must also be considered in any discussion of permanent expansion of coverage and long-term use of this service. Providers are typically paid significantly less for telehealth visits than for in-person visits. If telehealth payments remain well below those for the same services provided in person, that may create a financial disincentive that would make it difficult for providers to continue to offer telehealth services.

Navigating Payment Through Commercial Insurance

As described in the *Medicare Managed Care Manual,* MA plans must "provide their enrollees with all basic benefits covered under original Medicare. Consequently, plans may not impose limitations, waiting periods or exclusions from coverage due to pre-existing conditions that are not present in original Medicare." But for payment, the manual states, "MA plans need not follow original Medicare claims processing procedures. MA plans may create their own billing and payment procedures as long as providers—whether contracted or not—are paid accurately, timely and with an audit trail" (CMS, 2016). MA plans are also permitted to require enrollees to use contracted providers.

Unlike regular Medicare, where almost all inpatient admissions are paid on a DRG basis and outpatient services are paid by APC, commercial insurers pay hospitals in a variety of ways. These may include a per admission payment similar to a DRG, a payment for each day in the hospital (referred to as per diem payment), a payment for each hospital day which varies depending on where the patient receives services in the hospital, with a higher payment for intensive care and cardiac monitoring than for a routine medical/surgical unit, a set payment per service (similar to the APC method), and payment as a percentage of gross charges.

These payment methods can also vary between inpatient and outpatient care. For example, after careful analysis of insurance contracts, a hospital may determine that for several payers, they were paid more if a patient had knee replacement surgery as an outpatient (because the hospital was paid a percent of charges) than as an inpatient (where the hospital received a fixed payment). This example demonstrates that although inpatient admission is often preferable to outpatient care, payment may matter more than status.

In addition to a myriad of payment structures for providers, it is very difficult to estimate their financial obligations when they are hospitalized. Because of rising healthcare costs, more employers are offering the option of a high-deductible health plan, which has lower premiums but higher deductibles. As a result, the patient may owe 10%–50% of the costs of care, even after the deductible has been met, although the ability to set up a health savings account allows them to pay such liabilities with pre-tax dollars. MA plans also offer a variety of copayments, coinsurances, and deductibles.

Just as CMS has set up a variety of mandatory and optional bundled payment programs, so have commercial insurers. For example, in some areas of the country, insurers pay a fixed price to cover all care for cancer patients or for patients having elective joint or spine surgery (UnitedHealthcare, 2016). These programs are offered to self-insured employers and to select providers with a proven track record of quality and safety. Because insurers pay a fixed price, providers become responsible for determining how much they will be paid under these models. UnitedHealthcare reported savings of $10,000 or more per patient because of this program (Rudavsky, 2017). Some large employers, such as Walmart, are also contracting directly with select hospitals for such programs and are incentivizing their employees to travel to these centers by waiving all out-of-pocket costs and paying for all travel and expenses for a caregiver (Walmart, 2021).

How Physicians Are Paid

Unlike payments to hospitals, most payments to physicians are generally made on a fee-for-service basis, where increased volume leads to increased revenue. In general, physicians bill for two types of professional services: cognitive and procedural. The cognitive services are also referred to as evaluation and management (E/M) services and represent the office, clinic, or hospital visit by the physician where no procedure is performed. The procedural billing is for procedures, surgeries, or testing performed on the patient.

E/M services are generally billed based on the visit's complexity and the time that the patient spent with the physician. CMS has a confusing pair of coding guidelines—one from 1995 and one from 1997—that are both in use and are supposed to help a provider choose the proper E/M code for the visit. There are different E/M codes for different settings and different types of patient status, and each of the code ranges has levels of service based on the types of decision-making and examinations performed. For hospital visits, there are three codes to choose from for the first visit of the hospital stay, another three codes for subsequent visits, and two codes for services on the day of discharge. For office visits, there are four codes for new patient visits and a different set of five codes for established patient visits. CMS has defined a new patient as one who has not been seen by the physician or by any of their associates of the same specialty within the past three years.

To add to the confusion, in 2021, CMS adopted a new set of criteria for choosing the visit level for outpatient office visit E/M codes based on either time or the medical decision-making involved in the visit. The guidelines are expected to be expanded to all physician E/M services in 2023, but until that time, physicians providing non-outpatient office E/M services must use the criteria that best suits the site of service and the status of the patient. For instance, a cardiologist seeing a hospital outpatient receiving observation services would use the new outpatient visit guidelines to choose a code in the 99202–99215 range, whereas the hospitalist who orders the observation service would use the old guidelines to choose a code in the 99218–99220 range.

Procedural coding is based on the procedure(s) performed, and modifiers are appended to these codes to note unusual circumstances, such as complex cases, use of assistants, or cases terminated prior to completion. CMS assigns a global period to each procedure, which indicates the number of days after the procedure for which the physician cannot bill for additional visits unless there are extenuating circumstances. This global period is either zero days, 10 days, or 90 days.

This disconnect between the way physicians are paid (per service) and the way hospitals are paid (per admission) leads to a clash of incentives. Hospital leaders want the length of stay to be as short as is safe, whereas physicians may want to extend the stay so they can bill for more visits.

In 2007, CMS began to tie quality of care to physician reimbursement by paying physicians additional money for reporting their performance on certain quality measures (CMS, 2007). Initially, the Physician Quality Improvement Initiative, later renamed the Physician Quality Payment System, was a "pay for reporting" situation, as there was no quality threshold that had to be reached to receive added payment, and physicians instead received additional payments based on simply reporting quality measures. This approach was taken to gain physician buy-in and help physicians become comfortable with reporting such data. The program then developed into what is now the Merit-based Incentive Payment System (MIPS) (CMS, 1 November 2017). In MIPS, physicians must report data on quality measures and also complete practice improvement activities in order to score above a certain threshold and avoid a reduction in their payments from Medicare. To promote participation in alternative payment models such as ACOs, physicians who participate in those models are not required to report MIPS data, and they receive the maximum added payment allowable.

References

American Hospital Association. (November 2019). ICD-10-CM coding for social determinants of health. Retrieved from *aha.org/system/files/2018-04/value-initiative-icd-10-code-social-determinants-of-health.pdf*.

Bensken, W., Alberti, P. M., Koroukian, S.M. (May 2021). Health related social needs and increased readmission rates: Findings from the nationwide readmissions database. *Journal of General Internal Medicine, 36*(5): 1173–1180.

Centers for Medicare & Medicaid Services. (CMS). (10 August 2007). PRQI fact sheet. Retrieved from *https://www.cms.gov/Medicare/Quality-Initiatives-Patient-Assessment-Instruments/PQRS/downloads/2007_pqri_fact_sheet.pdf*.

CMS. (19 July 2013). CMS-1601-P. Retrieved from *https://www.cms.gov/Medicare/Medicare-Fee-for-Service-Payment/HospitalOutpatientPPS/Hospital-Outpatient-Regulations-and-Notices-Items/CMS-1601-P.html*.

CMS. (5 April 2013). Revision of Common Working File (CWF) editing for same-day, same- provider acute care readmissions. Retrieved from *https://www.cms.gov/Outreach-and-Education/Medicare-Learning-Network-MLN/MLNMattersArticles/downloads/MM3389.pdf*.

CMS. (6 May 2014). Three-day payment window. Retrieved from *https://www.cms.gov/Medicare/Medicare-Fee-for-Service-Payment/AcuteInpatientPPS/Three_Day_Payment_Window.html*.

CMS. (14 June 2014). Frequently asked questions CR 7502. Retrieved from *https://www.cms.gov/Medicare/Medicare-Fee-for-Service-Payment/AcuteInpatientPPS/Downloads/CR7502-FAQ.pdf*.

CMS. (22 April 2016). Chapter 4: Benefits and beneficiary protections. *Medicare Managed Care Manual.* Retrieved from *https://www.cms.gov/Regulations-and-Guidance/Guidance/Manuals/Downloads/mc86c04.pdf*.

CMS. (6 December 2017). Bundled Payments for Care Improvement (BPCI) initiative: General information. Retrieved from *https://innovation.cms.gov/initiatives/bundled-payments/*.

CMS. (22 December 2017). Comprehensive Care for Joint Replacement Model. Retrieved from *https://innovation.cms.gov/initiatives/cjr*.

CMS. (19 May 2017). Medicare program; Advancing care coordination through episode payment models (EPMs). *Federal Register.* Retrieved from h*ttps://www.federalregister.gov/documents/2017/05/19/2017-10340/medicare-program-advancing-care-coordination-through-episode-payment-models-epms-cardiac.*

CMS. (1 November 2017). Participation options overview. Retrieved from *https://qpp.cms.gov/mips/overview.*

CMS. (30 November 2017). Hospital Readmissions Reduction Program. Retrieved from *https://www.cms.gov/medicare/medicare-fee-for-service-payment/acuteinpatientpps/readmissions-reduction-program.html.*

CMS. (May 2021). Comprehensive Care for Joint Replacement model three-year extension and changes to episode definition and pricing. Retrieved from *https://www.federalregister.gov/documents/2021/05/03/2021-09097/medicare-program-comprehensive-care-for-joint-replacement-model-three-year-extension-and-changes-to.*

CMS. (2020). ICD-10-CM Official Guidelines for Coding and Reporting. Retrieved 10 June 2021 from *https://www.cms.gov/Medicare/Coding/ICD10/Downloads/2016-ICD-10-CM-Guidelines.pdf.*

Rau, J. (2 November 2020). Medicare fines half of hospitals for readmitting too many patients. Kaiser Health News. *https://khn.org/news/medicare-fines-half-of-hospitals-for-readmitting-too-many-patients/.*

Rudavsky, S. (13 January 2017). Bundled payments aim to control costs. Indystar.com. Retrieved from *https://www.indystar.com/story/money/2017/01/13/bundled-payments-aim-control-health-costs/96420390/.*

UnitedHealthcare. (1 December 2016). UnitedHealthcare launches new, value-based care payment to help improve health outcomes and reduce costs for knee, hip and spine procedures. Retrieved from *https://www.uhc.com/news-room/2016-news-release-archive/spine-and-joint-solution.*

Walmart. (June 2021). Walmart Centers of Excellence. Retrieved from *https://one.walmart.com/content/dam/themepage/pdfs/centers-of-excellence-2019.pdf.*

Yongkang, Z, Zhang Y, Sholle, E. (2020). Assessing the impact of social determinants of health on predictive models for potential avoidable 30-day readmission or death. Public Library of Science (PLOS) doi: 10.1371/journal.pone.0235064.

CHAPTER 4

Utilization Review Services

UR Is a Specialty Designation

Change doesn't come easy in hospitals and health systems, but this is even more the case when a change is systemic and far-reaching—precisely the intention of value-based care. New payment schemes turn the business model for hospitals upside down. In the past, hospital executives focused on putting "heads in beds" and providing services that generate income. Now under value-based care contracts, they're incentivized to keep people out of the hospital and only provide services that are clearly necessary. Additionally, executives have seen digital companies expand their footprint into primary and urgent care as consumers and providers became more comfortable with virtual care. Walmart Health, for example, is growing because their transparent pricing strategy and convenience of evening and weekend services make it an attractive alternative to hospital-based services. Amazon has entered the virtual primary care space by partnering with Care Medical, a private medical practice, and is promoting home-based care for chronic care patients and post-acute care management. These companies may pose some financial threat to hospitals and health systems that remain entrenched in traditional models and resist the movement to value-based care and patient convenience.

Once hospital executives embrace changes to their traditional business model, operational challenges will arise. As hospital leaders seek to maximize the effectiveness of clinical operations to overcome the traditional silos of care, they will find success in a value-based environment by achieving "systemness," a word used to describe hospital staff who seek greater cooperation and interaction between multiple service areas to improve coordination. As an example, the move to regionalize hospitalists has reduced the travel time physicians spend traipsing from one medical unit to another and has contributed to greater team collaboration. It has also led to the creation of accountable care units, which raise the bar on care coordination and appropriate use of resources.

Hospital case management programs are not immune to these transformative dynamics. Although many hospitals are still using the once-popular 1990s model of combining discharge planning and utilization review (UR), others are shifting to care coordination models as the organization prepares for value-based care, population health, or a new accountable care organization where care and services for vulnerable patient populations will be coordinated across the entire continuum. As a result, a new emphasis has been placed on the organization and intent of case management programs resulting in realignment of care coordination and UR activities and changes in reporting structure and operations. The UR role is finally, and deservedly, becoming a distinct specialty worthy of the attention being given to it by the senior executive team and, most importantly, the chief financial officer (CFO).

The UR specialist

Before the introduction of the prospective payment system (PPS), nurses performed perfunctory UR activities. Many hospitals believed that registered nurses (RN) were suited for this role based on their ability to communicate with the physicians and the payers at a time when "reasonable and necessary" medical interventions were largely left to the prerogative of the physician (*Social Security Act §1862*). Who better to interpret physicians' intentions—and handwriting—than a nurse?

The PPS' fixed rate methodology, introduced in 1983, created an incentive to be more frugal with hospital resources. If expenses exceeded the fixed rate that the Centers for Medicare & Medicaid Services (CMS) paid, the hospital would lose money. If expenses were less than the fixed payment rate, the hospital would have a positive margin. But a problem arose when, instead of focusing on the expenses associated with the use of resources in caring for the patient, hospital executives became absorbed in reducing length of stay (LOS). There was an assumption, still held by many hospital executives, that reducing LOS would result in significant cost reduction. However, this approach did not work. A 1986 study in New Jersey confirmed that "the [cost reduction] incentives attributed to the diagnosis-related groupings (DRG) concept did not have a differential impact." This was the first objective indication that reductions in LOS did not yield a concomitant reduction in costs (Hsiao, Sapolsky, Dunn, and Weiner, 1986). While LOS may be a worthy metric to evaluate operational efficiency, and it certainly impacts risk of infection and patient safety, subsequent studies have challenged the pervasive belief that hospital costs can be significantly curtailed by reducing LOS (Tahari, Butz, and Greenfield, 2000).

By the early 1990s, executives in the hospitals that survived the post-DRG financial chaos saw that more drastic measures had to be taken to reduce costs, and the era of hospital reengineering began. An early success story took place at New England Medical Center (NEMC), where hospital leaders were able to reduce LOS *and* associated costs by redesigning the nursing delivery model. The redesign introduced the concept of hospital case management in which the admitting nurses figuratively took off their clinical caps and put on their case management hats. They followed selected patients in the role as the patients' case manager while those patients moved through the acute care episode. Their role included coordination with patients' new care teams, as the nurse "case manager" updated the new care team about the patient's treatment plan, the patient's response to the plan, the tests that were completed, the tests that were outstanding, and other information sharing that would expedite progression of care and result in lowering LOS.

As hospital management engineers slashed and burned extraneous positions and consolidated processes to reduce hospital costs, they tried to emulate the NEMC model and created a new department called case management. The case management department combined and reduced the number of full-time employees previously budgeted for social work and UR. However, the basic tenet of care coordination as practiced at NEMC got lost. Instead, the staff from the previous UR department continued to perform UR functions, and the social workers took on broadened discharge planning roles in what's been characterized as functional case management models, as noted in *The Hospital Case Management Orientation Manual* by Peggy Rossi, BSN, MPA, CCM, and Karen Zander, RN, MS, CMAC, FAAN.

Variations of this functional model still exist today, as case managers perform UR in many hospitals as well as discharge planning, and social service departments have mostly disappeared. But the release of the 1999 Institute of Medicine report "To Err Is Human" signaled the beginning of a new marketplace that called for dramatic improvements in hospital quality and safety outcomes. Progressive case management leaders and their executive sponsors used the opportunity to rethink case management goals as originally reintroduced and create new models. As a result, teams of specialists schooled in the rules and regulations governing UR in the private and public sector took on UR functions.

Today, UR specialists occupy center stage in the hospital's effort to effectively monitor acute care medical necessity so that acute care services are reserved for those with acute care needs. They serve in access management departments to work with the admissions and bed management staff to review acute level of care appropriateness as part of the pre-registration/registration processes for direct admits and inter- and intra-hospital transfers. They work in the emergency department (ED) alongside the physicians and nurses and serve as real-time advisors to the clinical team about documenting acute medical necessity. They are also seen on the hospital units to speak with the nurses and care coordinators and share information with the hospitalists and community physicians, who often look to their expertise to make decisions about the continuing need for acute level of care or discharge readiness. Some also work remotely from centralized office spaces or from home, where electronic access to the patient's medical record makes it convenient to perform continued-stay reviews.

Professional nurses continue to dominate the field of first-level UR, but licensed practical nurses have gained a foothold in the area, especially in communities where professional nurse resources are scarce. Other disciplines with keen knowledge of medical terminology, such as emergency medical technicians or clinical documentation integrity (CDI) specialists, are also being enlisted, especially with the presence of the electronic health record (EHR) and information found in the nationally recognized guidelines, such as Hearst's MCG Care Guidelines or Change Healthcare's InterQual®. The guidelines, together with the medical documentation, serve as the source of the UR specialist's suggestions to the physician. And when they are available electronically, it generally takes the guessing out of the first-level screening process, allowing for a broader—and possibly less costly—assortment of backgrounds within the UR specialist workforce.

Job Descriptions and Performance Expectations

UR specialists are found in hospitals of just about every size. They often hold part-time positions in small critical access hospitals (CAH) and may serve as on-call resources. CAHs or small community hospitals may not need a full-time team to oversee compliance with the *Conditions of Participation (CoP)* and to influence medical necessity decisions, but a UR specialist's expert knowledge can be a valuable asset at any time. Unless these small hospitals are financially or statutorily concerned about complying with CMS or contractual medical necessity requirements—which may benefit from a real-time coaching resource working with the medical staff—they often outsource the function to another organization or use an external community agency approved by CMS.

The value and benefits of having a dedicated UR specialist working in real time with the medical staff, physician advisor (PA), and care coordinator team cannot be overstated. UR specialists are always an asset as long as they are experts in what they do and proficient in how they do it. Proficiency is key: Every UR specialist must accurately complete a review of medical documentation for medical necessity and recommend a level of care based on the documentation and criteria being used. In addition, the specialist must critically review the completeness of the physician's documentation to ensure that it will withstand the scrutiny of oversight agencies and payers. It is no longer sufficient to find the key words that fulfill the criteria. Rather, the UR specialist must be able to offer an opinion about whether the physician's documentation supports the criteria and portrays a concise picture of the severity of the patient's needs at the time of admission. Cases are at risk for payment denial even if elements fulfilling the criteria are present, unless the documentation accurately portrays a complete picture of the patient's status that conjures up the patient's condition far distant from current presentation. The payer's reviewing physician will use the medical narrative to gain a clear understanding of why the patient was admitted to the hospital even if the review is occurring six months or a year following the patient's discharge.

Inter-rater reliability testing, a qualitative rating process that defines the degree of agreement between multiple UR specialists, can allow the experienced UR specialist to objectively measure proficiency in documentation review and application of criteria. If UR specialists are appropriately educated in the use of the hospital's guidelines and the rules of medical necessity documentation, then each one should have the same answers as colleagues. An annual rating of less than 92% should be grounds for reeducation and may lead to dismissal of an individual if his or her performance does not improve. Oversight agencies and payers are looking over every provider's shoulder, which means that no organization should permit less-than-stellar performance by those who are the first line of defense in maintaining revenue integrity and reducing hospital-associated patient risk.

What makes a successful UR specialist candidate?

We frequently get asked the question of what makes a successful UR specialist candidate, but over the years, we have found that there is no single answer that encapsulates the perfect candidate. However, there are several common requisites. Among the most essential characteristics are confidence and assertive communication skills. Specifically, the UR specialist must be able to leverage his or her clinical knowledge to evaluate whether the documentation demonstrating the patient's severity of illness and prescribed treatment plan coupled with the guidelines in use warrants a hospital level of care. Although nationally recognized criteria can guide a decision on medical necessity, the UR specialist will use the content of the physician's documentation to support the admitting physician's determination of appropriate status.

The assertive UR specialist speaks up if any aspect of a case seems curious, which frequently means guiding emergency department physicians in their decisions about the most appropriate status or the attending physician's decision about his or her patients' need for continuing care. It means questioning a decision and bringing up issues that were not considered or addressed. If UR specialists are going to be in the position of questioning or coaching members of the medical staff, they had better be secure in their level of knowledge and skills so they can withstand probable pushback, which many physicians will exercise until they feel confident in the UR specialist's advice.

The successful candidate works with a healthy curiosity and a well-honed knowledge of basic clinical information and medical jargon and a sound familiarity with a regulatory landscape that seems to shift weekly. The work often involves situations and settings in which the specialist is forced to give advice with which he or she may not personally agree. For example, a UR specialist may feel that, on compassionate grounds, a patient should have access to a particular treatment or medication, but that service may not be covered due to the specifics of the case, hospital policy, or the terms of the insurance policy. The UR specialist will need to clarify that such treatment is not covered regardless of his or her personal feelings.

Credentials

Like their care coordinator colleagues, UR specialists come from a variety of clinical backgrounds. Although the vast majority are nurses in all stages of their careers, many successful UR specialists come with knowledge grounded in physical therapy, pharmacy, or other clinical specialties. In geographic areas of scarce resources, licensed practical nurses and emergency medical technicians are ably filling the roles. At the present time, unfortunately, there is not a credential specific to UR. However, the following credentials are available if you qualify.

The American Board of Quality Assurance and Utilization Review Physicians (ABQAURP) offers a credential in Health Care Quality and Management (HCQM). (See *www.abqaurp.org.*)

The National Board of Prior Authorization Specialists offers certification as a PACS—Prior Authorization Certified Specialist. It is a self-paced online education program for allied health workers and admissions/access management personnel who regularly work with payers. (See *www.priorauthtraining.org.*)

To become a Certified Managed Care Nurse, candidates must hold an RN license or a license in practical nursing in any American state, territory, or protectorate. To become a Certified Managed Care Professional (CMCP), candidates for the CMCP credential must hold a valid social worker license or license in professional counseling. The CMCP exam covers components such as managed care overview, healthcare economics, healthcare management, and patient issues. The exam is administered by the American Board of Managed Care Nursing (see *ABMCN.org* for details).

Although there are basic expectations of a UR team member, organizations should develop performance expectations and competencies for their UR staff based on their own needs (see Figure 4.1 for a sample job description).

■ **Figure 4.1**

Utilization review specialist job description

I. Job description:

Conduct medical certification review for medical necessity for acute care facility and services. Use nationally recognized, evidence-based guidelines approved by medical staff in conjuction with medical documentation to recommend level of care to the physician and serve as a resource to the medical staff on issues related to admission qualifications, resource utilization, national and local coverage determinations, and documentation improvement opportunities.

II. Eligibility requirements:

- Graduate of a practical or professional school of nursing with licensure, or eligible for licensure, as an LPN or RN in the state. Other disciplines or comparable experience will be considered.
- Expert knowledge of InterQual® Level of Care Criteria or MCG and knowledge of local and national coverage determinations.
- Recent work experience in the hospital or insurance industry.
- Eligibility to remain in this position requires an annual 92% proficiency rating based on objective inter-rater reliability testing.

Utilization review specialist job description (cont.)

III. Precertification:

- Collaborates with the access management team to provide accurate and complete clinical information in order to obtain precertification/authorization.

- Reviews operating room (OR) schedule 48 hours in advance of scheduled procedures to confirm that all eligible Medicare and Medicaid admissions were identified, a pre-authorization was obtained as necessary, and the coded procedure is or is not on the Medicare inpatient-only list. Confirms that physician's admission orders accurately reflect status.

- Reviews medical documents of all elective, direct, and transfer patient requests prior to patient's arrival to confirm medical necessity and level of care. If documentation does not adequately support patient's need for hospital level of care and the admitting physician is resistant to advice, the case is promptly referred to the physician advisor (PA) for remediation.

- Consistently completes the transfer agreement between the hospital and the transferring facility, and advises the inpatient care manager of expected length of stay.

IV. Access to care:

- Conducts inpatient pre-admission and admission review for Medicare and Medicaid beneficiaries as well as private insurance members and self-pay patients based on CMS guidelines and specific payer contract requirements.

- Pre-admission and admission reviews are done concurrently at the point of entry in collaboration with ED and admitting physician and the cooperation with the access management team to determine the appropriateness of hospital level of care.

- Confers with ED and admitting physicians when documentation does not appear to support inpatient status and offers suggestions for clarity and completeness.

- Uses InterQual Level of Care Criteria or MCG to screen for appropriateness for inpatient status or observation services based on physician documentation, H&P, treatment plan, potential risks, and basis for expectation of a two-midnight stay.

- Understands and applies federal law regarding the use of Hospital Initiated Notice of Non-Coverage (HINN), Medicare Outpatient Observation Notice (MOON), and Advance Beneficiary Notice (ABN) for all applicable patients.

- Ensures that commercial payers are immediately advised if their members do not qualify for inpatient status according to criteria used.

- Keeps current on all regulatory changes that affect delivery or reimbursement of acute care services. Uses knowledge of national and local coverage determinations to appropriately advise physicians.

- Proactively confers with admitting physician to provide coaching on accurate status and level of care determination at point-of-hospital entry.

- Consistently identifies and records information on any progression-of-care/patient flow barriers.

- Consults with medical staff, care team, and case managers as necessary to resolve immediate progression-of-care barriers through appropriate administrative and medical channels.

- Engages care team colleagues in collaborative problem-solving regarding appropriate utilization of resources.

- Promotes the use of best practice guidelines at point-of-entry and notes any undocumented deviations.

- Collaborates with community physicians and hospitalists to influence appropriate utilization of resources, accurate status determination, and transitions of care.

- Recognizes and responds appropriately to patient safety/risk factors.

V. Continuing stay:

- Actively participates in daily huddles, multidisciplinary rounds, patient care conferences, and hospitalist/nurse handoff reports to maintain knowledge about intensity of services and the progression of care.

Utilization review specialist job description (cont.)

- Identifies potentially wasteful or misused resources and recommends alternatives if appropriate by analyzing clinical protocols.
- Maintains appropriate documentation on each patient to include specific information of all resource utilization activities.
- Ensures that a long-stay certification signed by the attending physician is recorded in the medical record by day 20 and alerts the physician or case manager to resolve.
- Identifies and records episodes of preventable delays or avoidable days due to failure of progression-of-care processes.
- Educates members of the patient's care team on the appropriate access to and use of various levels of care.
- Represents utilization management at various committees, professional organizations, and physician groups as needed.
- Promotes use of evidence-based protocols and/or order sets to influence high-quality and cost-effective care.
- Promotes medical documentation that accurately reflects findings and interventions, presence of complications or comorbidities, quality and safety indicators, and patient's need for continuing stay.
- Proactively participates as a member of the interdisciplinary clinical team to confirm appropriateness of the treatment plan relative to the patient's preference, reason for admission, and availability of resources.
- Confers with attending physician and PA if medically unnecessary inpatient treatment is contemplated. Issues the appropriate HINN if not resolved.

VI. Transition:

- Confirms patient's readiness for discharge based on medical necessity for continued acute care stay
- Consults with the patient's nurse to confirm agreement by the patient and the care team concerning the discharge plan
- Opens a communication channel with post-acute services arranged through the resource center to stay current on finding and arranging services to initiate discharge plan
- Serves as a resource person to physicians, case managers, physician offices, and billing office for coverage and compliance issues
- Works closely with decision support personnel to review resource utilization data and trends to identify outliers who may benefit from real-time coaching to improve outcomes

Source: Phoenix Medical Management, Inc., in Pompano Beach, Florida. Adapted with permission.

Staffing the UR Team

How should the UR team be staffed? Without a doubt, this is the number one question we are asked by hospital clients. It would be great if we had the magic answer. Unfortunately, there are no best practice standards, as the answer depends on the individual organization and several variables. Informal productivity benchmarks estimate that reviewers spend 20–30 minutes on each continuing stay case. This may help organizations calculate the time spent on reviews and thereby determine how many reviewers are needed, but there are no hard and fast rules or specific guidelines. Program leaders and executive sponsors should also use caution when considering the use of data from productivity metric sources or professional UR associations, as the statistics often do not consider all the variables existing in the reporting facilities. In addition, many of the popular productivity applications used by human resources and finance leaders may place UR full-time employees into productivity slots that are not related to job expectations. It is not unusual, for example, to discover UR staff members grouped with social workers in some popular productivity benchmark applications. Combining these two different types of professionals in the same group will not provide reliable data, and benchmarks and will result in skewed expectations. If external reports are used to evaluate staffing, ensure these reports are comparing apples to apples.

■ **Figure 4.2**

Staffing variables	
VARIABLE	**CONSIDERATION**
Payer mix	Regular Medicare versus commercial volumes and alternative payment models.
State Medicaid requirements	Whether regular Medicaid or managed Medicaid, each state may have specific review and data entry requirements. Many states are now using dedicated software applications, which can be burdensome due to the amount of time it takes to process reviews.
Contract language	Boilerplate cooperation puts the UR specialist in a defensive posture subject to the demands of the payer reviewers. Specific expectations via negotiated addendum will speed up the process.
Current payer expectations	Is the UR specialist expected to "regurgitate" the contents of the medical record documents or just provide pertinent positives?
Denial experience	Percent of actual EDI 835 remittances that are completely or partially denied or denied pending more information.
Scope of UR specialist practice	Other responsibilities may include presumptive audits, capture of delays and CDI, case appeals, and readmission review.
Admission sources	Percent of patients coming from the ED, direct admits, and inter-hospital or intra-hospital transfers.
Presence of on-site payer reviewers	Avoid duplication of effort between hospital and payer UR specialist, but make sure that the contract protects the hospital in the case of concurrent denials.
Payer access to HIPAA-compliant portal	Avoid duplication of effort, but make sure that the contract protects the hospital in the case of concurrent denials.
Content of the EHR	Full EHR versus hybrid records (a combination of paper and electronic).
Skill level	New recruits versus seasoned; proficiency scores.
Electronic resources	Access to interactive UR system versus online version of criteria sets or paper manual to be referenced.
Teaching or non-teaching facility	Affects the volume of medical documents that must be reviewed.

Source: Phoenix Medical Management, Inc., in Pompano Beach, Florida. Reprinted with permission.

UR specialists are generally on-site seven days a week, though there are many organizations with remote staff who, following best practices, manage most of the pre-admits and continued-stay reviews. However, the one commonality among the vast majority of hospitals is the presence of a UR specialist in the ED. As

UR shifts from a clinical activity to a revenue cycle activity, the value of placing UR specialists in the ED increases because they can establish proactive, real-time processes working directly with the admitting physicians. Ensuring that UR specialists are available in the ED seven days a week helps spread out the volume of work and avoids Monday morning backlogs of activities that need follow-up. This proactive, front-end revenue cycle–focused strategy establishes a real-time gatekeeping process and is in contrast to older UR models that placed the function in a reactive and retrospective position, reviewing patients only after they were a "head in a bed," and too often focusing resources on frustrating attempts to find back-end fixes.

Hospital financial leaders find that having a resource available to the admitting physicians is a core component of a successful front-end revenue cycle and is easily quantifiable as a return on investment. In fact, if UR resources are limited in your facility, the best way to optimize those scarce assets would be to have a UR specialist attached to the ED or colocated between the ED and other access management services, such as pre-admits and transfers.

UR Specialists and the Medical Staff

At a conference we attended not long ago, a UR specialist spoke about the daily challenges she experienced as a seasoned reviewer. "If I didn't have to deal with the doctors, my life would be a whole lot more pleasant," she said. We can all laugh at this statement, but in reality some physicians do present a challenge. Although this statement is not true for every physician, as a group, they can generate stress even among the most experienced reviewers. There are many reasons for this, but in general, it's because they have not been taught the nuances of UR or documentation. Unfortunately, universities do not offer courses such as "How to survive your first year as a medical resident," or "Everything I needed to know as a resident, I learned from a UR specialist." Therein lies the challenge; at teaching hospitals, the case management department, UR specialist team, chief compliance officer, or PA should provide educational programs on regulatory and accrediting agency requirements for physicians. If your organization doesn't do so, contact the teaching faculty sponsor and make it happen! Medical students, interns, and residents are sponges. They want to know the ins and outs of the healthcare industry, and the UR team should take advantage of this by offering education. Without formal education, residents will learn from each other—or worse, from the attending physicians—which is rarely optimal.

Hospitalists are also ripe for information, and 75% of hospitals now employ hospitalists (Page, 2016). Many hospitalists have incentive compensation packages that include outcomes related to documentation, readmissions, quality and safety indicators, and denial exposure. Sharing information on the rules governing medical necessity and teaching them to learn to document more accurately and completely will go a long way toward improving relationships and developing care teams whose members share mutual goals for exceptional patient care. Bear in mind that the UR team will also have to work with several generations that may have varying comfort levels when dealing with technology. More senior physicians may be less proficient; however, younger physicians who are more proficient may also be more likely to use shortcuts, such as copy and paste, that can adversely affect the accuracy of the medical record.

Community physicians present different UR challenges because they are not routinely present in the hospital. Their livelihood is heavily dependent on their office practice, so their time in the hospital must be structured and purposeful. They will likely resist any intrusion that they believe is peripheral to their primary goals of caring for their patients and quickly returning to their practices. Working with this group of physicians will require mature communication skills that convey a message of a value-added partnership. That partnership may be easier to establish in view of *Medicare Program Integrity Transmittal 541,* which was effective 8 September 2014 and gives the Medicare Administrative Contractor (MAC) and the Zone Program Integrity Contractor the discretion to automatically deny a Part B claim submitted by a proceduralist or surgeon if it is related to a Part A claim that has been denied for lack of medical necessity for the procedure or surgery. This adds leverage that neither the case managers nor UR specialists had in the past. Although this transmittal has not been applied to date, it illustrates CMS' intent to increasingly hold physicians responsible for their role in care that is determined to be not medically necessary. It remains to be seen if it is evoked as hospital and physician payments slowly shift to new models of reimbursement.

UR and CDI

Accurate clinical documentation is a vital component of patient care, physician satisfaction, and revenue cycle strategies. But CDI programs have not fundamentally changed to meet new marketplace demands since their introduction in 1992 by J.A. Thomas. The majority of CDI programs encountered by us focus on task-based activities with the use of customary, task-based key performance indicators (KPI), such as the number of charts reviewed, the number of queries left, physician query agreement rates, comorbidity or complication (CC)/major CC capture rate, etc. The CDI role, based on multiple job description reviews, confirms that supporting the coding process to attaining the appropriate DRG is a key expectation. These traditional programs "unrelentingly focus upon capturing and recording a diagnosis being managed for treatment" and overlook documentation "insufficiencies and shortcomings" that can affect communication and continuity of patient care while resulting in downstream repercussions (Krauss, 2017). They overlook the opportunity to enhance the value and completeness of the patient's story that is fundamental to the establishment of medical necessity to justify hospital level of care. Based on our interviews with CFOs, it appears that the executive team's ongoing support of this legacy CDI approach assumes that hitting KPI targets coupled with case-mix index increases represent a reliable measure of CDI effectiveness. But they neglect to consider the other side of the coin: the denials that pour in each month because documentation poorly represents the patient's need for hospital level of care or continuing stay and the back office costs of fixing the problems and resubmitting correct claims. The patient's medical record is the repository of the patient's story. Quality documentation—more complete, more accurate, and more concise—can accomplish multiple goals: demonstrate the severity of the patient's condition, the risk of mortality, and the overall clinical picture. At the same time, it should support the coded diagnoses and procedures. CDI programs should increase their value by focusing on both equally critical goals.

Baylor Scott & White Health recently escaped a False Claims whistleblower lawsuit alleging they up-coded claims through their CDI program. A Texas judge dismissed the lawsuit, saying there is nothing wrong with hospitals taking advantage of coding opportunities to increase Medicare payment that is supported by documentation. In fact, as CDI programs grew in popularity, CMS noted "we do not believe there is anything inappropriate, unethical, or otherwise wrong with hospitals taking full advantage of coding opportunities to maximize Medicare payment as long as the coding is fully and properly supported by documentation in the medical record" (Sullivan, 2020). However, Glenn Krauss, a recognized CDI expert, argues that "the [CDI] community is assuming that the language used to toss out the whistleblower lawsuit sanctions the misguided approach to CDI that has remained virtually stagnant for the past 12 years." His point is well taken when reports of the growing volume of first-pass payer denials, clinical validation denials, adverse level of care determinations, and DRG downgrades haunt the C-suite. CDI capture of additional diagnosis codes really "don't mean much in the telling of the patient's clinical story" (Krauss, 2019). Therefore, it is important UR specialists only make documentation suggestions to the physician that support the patient's story and explain the medical necessity of the assigned status or level of care.

In the persistent drive for operational efficiency, hospital leaders should consider the number of people who are reviewing the same documentation but have different focuses in mind. UR staff are trying to ensure that the patient status is correct and supported by the clarity of the medical documentation; CDI specialists are trying to promote documentation that contains greater specificity and reflects the patient's story in a correct, complete, and consistent manner; and medical record coders are reviewing the same series of documents to assign accurate codes for the claim forms and comply with the broad array of regulatory reporting requirements. There is some discussion that the introduction of the International Classification of Diseases 11th Revision (ICD-11) in 2022 may prompt an integrated approach to medical documentation by combining the CDI and UR role and linking the position to the coding process, due to the volume of codes in ICD-11 and the documentation that would be needed to defend coding decisions. Currently, coding, CDI, and UR do not always work closely together. There are benefits, even now, to bringing those functions closer together to create a coordinated, cohesive effort to ensure documentation in the medical record that supports patient status, level of care, accurate diagnoses, and correct coding. Perhaps it is time to review different revenue cycle integration models and consider how to tackle challenges across organizational boundaries.

The traditional, task-oriented models of CDI allow hospitals to optimize revenue under the current fee-for-service system and also provide a strong picture of the overall health of the population that will need care in value-based payment systems. Indeed, risk-adjusted payment methodologies rely heavily on historical data to predict healthcare costs based on the relative risk of the patient population. But once value-based payments expand across regions, the focus of metrics assessing provided care will shift more heavily to factors such as quality and clinical outcomes and cost savings. So, although a traditional CDI program provides valid data, as hospitals move to new payment methods, those traditional programs will have to shift to ensure that the content of the medical documentation is thorough, comprehensive, and entered in a timely fashion so that subsequent readers will understand what was provided and why it was provided. To paraphrase the title of this book, a "contemporary" CDI program should ensure quality clinical documentation as well as the data necessary for healthcare providers to meet the ongoing demands for validation of quality of care and lower costs.

In addition, physicians should realize that the only way their clinical performance is adjudicated by those outside of the hospital is through claims data, and claims data is a product of physician documentation and coding. A CDI/UR specialist is the perfect resource to use when learning what can impact the accuracy of reported data. If the billing data is incorrect, then physician performance will be adjudicated incorrectly.

MACRA, MIPS, and UR/CDI

The Medicare Access and CHIP Reauthorization Act (MACRA) permanently repealed the flawed sustainable growth rate that CMS had been using to determine physician payment rates each year. Without getting into details of how physicians get paid, suffice it to say that under MACRA, MIPS is one of two payment track options that physicians can choose. The process adjusts Medicare Part B payments based on performance in four performance categories: quality, cost, promoting interoperability, and improvement activities. As you can imagine, a lot of information used to determine these scores comes from claims data, which comes from documentation. Poor, inadequate documentation and the proliferation of copied and pasted documentation should be of particular concern to MIPS-participating physicians, as their revenue will depend upon their documentation skills.

At the same time, CDI programs are becoming more sophisticated as new applications for smartphones and tablets support CDI queries that are more focused on the significance of findings of exams and test results. These applications can track categories of documentation weaknesses to identify areas ripe for physician education. By streamlining the query and response process, coders will be able to shorten the time between review and dropping a clean bill.

Similarly, the introduction of computer-assisted coding (CAC) applications adds a new dimension to the role of the UR specialist. CAC uses technology and linguistics within the EHR to translate clinical language to ICD-10 Clinical Modification/Procedure Coding System, Current Procedural Terminology®, Systematized Nomenclature of Medicine, and other codes using mapping across these data standards. Some CAC applications can highlight key clinical terms in selected documents for easy recognition by reviewers and coders. CAC applications can auto-assign an ICD-10 code based on data entered, ensuring compliance with coding guidelines and enabling consistency in clinical documentation across clinicians.

CAC applications may also support concurrent coding that could result in reducing the coding staff and refocusing coders on using their acumen and experience to expand the UR/CDI team capacities. With additional positions, the time frame between patient discharge and claim preparation may be shortened, as well the time spent in accounts receivable.

Effectively integrating some or all primary review activities—UR, CDI, and concurrent coding—is a challenge and one with no best practice solution with which we are familiar. Defining the connection between these functions and developing practical processes that build on those connections are important issues that the healthcare industry must solve in the coming years.

Reporting Structure—Is It Finance, Compliance, or Case Management?

Healthcare transformation is dictated largely by new payment arrangements that reward value and include varying degrees of shared risk. The resulting changes are often accompanied by an escalating administrative burden of policies, rules, and regulations that determine hospital and medical staff payment. It is important to have a well-informed team of revenue and regulatory specialists who can use their knowledge of access to care requirements, regulatory specifics, quality improvement organizations, accrediting agency standards, inpatient and outpatient eligibility, and contractual requirements. These specialists must also understand the concept of prior authorization and how it affects length of stay to protect the physicians, patients, and hospital against the financial risks associated with new payment obligations.

In general, hospitals posted a median operating margin of only 0.3% in 2020, although with funding from the CARES Act, the margin was 2.7% (Kaufman Hall, 2021). Although 2020 was an unusual year, hospital cost drivers kept pumping with investments in new technology, higher salaries and benefit expenses, and higher supply and drug costs. But estimates show that upwards of $33.7 billion of hospital costs result from potentially avoidable admissions (McDermot and Jiang, 2020), $39 billion result from the delay or refusal to use evidence-based treatment protocols (IMS, 2013), $130 billion stem from inefficiently delivered services (Institute of Medicine, 2010), and $7.42 million are due to intensive care unit (ICU) transfer delays (Bagshaw et al., 2020).

Opportunities to reduce costs through tight management of access and continued-stay necessity provide a compelling business case for aligning UR activities with the revenue cycle team and revenue integrity programs. Indeed, there seems to be a mini-trend in this direction. Informal feedback to us from UR specialists who work under this reporting structure report they receive more relevant information pertaining to their specialty than they did under prior leaders and in a more timely manner.

On the other hand, we have encountered hospitals whose leaders see utilization management activities as part of the hospital's obligation to comply with the *CoP*, especially those sections relating to medical necessity reviews for admissions, continued stay, and professional services (CMS, 2011). They also view UR specialists as the first line of defense against any deviation from the rules and regulations governing Medicare participation, such as compliance with patient notices. Depending upon the size of the facility, a hospital may have someone acting as the chief compliance officer (CCO), a dedicated CCO, or, as in larger hospitals or integrated delivery systems, an Office of Compliance and Business Conduct. The scope of responsibilities also reflects the size of the facility, but in facilities greater than 200 beds, the key functions of the compliance officer include upholding compliance with all applicable laws, regulations, and standards. It is not unusual for the compliance office to house an internal audit staff that is constantly auditing, testing, and reeducating staff on the hospital's compliance program. Without that diligence, it can be easy to miss or to fail to uncover a system defect or unintentional fraud. Oversight agencies such as CMS, the Office of Inspector General (OIG), and the Department of Justice (DOJ) do not look kindly on hospital executives who fail to discover and remedy noncompliant practices, especially those related to the *CoP*, coding, and billing.

Finally, there are organizations where UR activities remain integrated within the case management program. In these models, the case manager is typically responsible for creating and implementing every patient's discharge plan and is expected to perform UR activities. This legacy model was cited in the Case Management Society of America's White Paper on Hospital Case Management Practice as one that "detracts from the case managers' practice standard obligation and the related opportunities which this era of value-based care demands" (CMSA, 2019). In addition, these outdated models often result in the insurer assigning their care coordinators to work around the hospital staff and monitor resource utilization, timely progression of care, and discharge for their selected high-risk members. This often results in communication gaps as well as tension between the two competing roles. Alternatively, these programs may have taken the first step toward distinguishing care coordination from utilization review and separated the two functions while remaining together structurally. These joint models are often under the executive sponsorship of the chief medical officer, chief operating officer, vice president of medical affairs, lead hospitalist, and occasionally the chief nursing officer.

Inter-Professional Communication

Effective communication methods must be established regardless of which UR model the hospital chooses. Even in the older functional models where one person (typically a case manager) may be doing both discharge planning and UR, the information gathered must be shared with other members of the care team—a requisite for effective care coordination. If a UR team is carved out from the case management program and reports to finance or compliance, communication with other members of the care team may pose a greater challenge.

The literature is filled with articles and case studies demonstrating that communication and teamwork are essential for providing quality healthcare. Teams that span the professional boundaries can capitalize on the variety of knowledge, skills, and abilities available to influence care and patient safety. In 2015, the Risk Management Foundation of Harvard's Medical Institute reported that the average indemnity payment of $484,000 was due to provider-to-provider communication gaps. Consequently, professional organizations continue to emphasize the importance of teamwork training in the delivery of safe care and sharing critical patient information. Every member of the hospital care team must work collaboratively with their peers to accomplish shared goals within and across settings to achieve coordinated, high-quality care. Yet barriers to teamwork are persistent, probably because the training of healthcare professionals is generally isolated by discipline, which can result in varying norms and values and thus impedes the development of shared knowledge, skills, and attitudes. As David Nash, MD, founding dean emeritus at Jefferson College of Population Health, explained, "team-based care is foreign to many physicians who were trained to lead themselves, not others" (Betbeze, 2013). It also could be that hospitals have long-standing operational silos that make inter-professional communication an extremely difficult endeavor.

It is unfortunate that neither new hospital associates nor medical students, interns, and residents are schooled in the requirements of UR nor provided any onboarding information regarding regulatory requirements. As a result, attempts to communicate with them may be met by pushback or only a perfunctory acknowledgment of the UR specialist's review findings. These barriers interfere with the organization's expectation of collaborative care efforts and derail its ability to leverage each discipline's professional strengths to effectively manage throughput. Throughput obstacles are well known to the UR specialist and case managers but are rarely quantified for their financial impact nor reviewed by the UR committee despite persistent C-suite complaints about throughput obstacles.

It is ultimately the responsibility of hospital executives to remove barriers to communication and implement policies and culture changes that foster a team approach that emphasizes everyone's duty to support patient care and manage potential financial risks to patients and the hospital. This can be accomplished in part by creating greater clarity on roles and expectations and enforcing core teamwork competencies, including leadership, situation monitoring, mutual support, and communication. Hospital executives may hold formal, multidisciplinary meetings to advance these goals. If communication and teamwork are not supported at the executive level and the executives do not give clear signals that they support UR, the UR team will not be able to realize its critical goals of improving oversight and reducing financial and quality risks, such as poor documentation of medical necessity.

The general communication and teamwork principles that must be established for the UR program and clinical departments overall must also be applied to specific functions and tasks, such as medical necessity reviews. The specific structure and form of communication for UR activities will vary based on the hospital's UR model. If the facility maintains a portion of the patient's medical record on paper, more in-person communication may be necessary, since the UR specialist must be able to access the charts on the patient care units. In those hospitals, the UR specialist is regularly accessible and often more visible to the hospitalists, case managers, and members of the patient's clinical team. Some hospitals experimenting with accountable care units (ACU) may assign a UR specialist with one or more care coordinators to work with the ACU team. Other hospitals assign UR specialists to medical specialties or medical groups that are large admitters. It is important to select the right model for the particular setting rather than taking a one-size-fits-all approach. For example, unit-based models outside of ACUs don't work as well because patients are often moved to other units and continuity of UR oversight suffers. Program leaders often opt to assign UR specialists by payer with the anticipation that the relationship the UR specialist builds with the payer's counterpart will benefit the facility. This is also very popular in hospitals using a virtual model; the UR specialist team may be physically centralized on or off campus, but they are assigned to specific payers.

A solid communication system is necessary as UR specialists become more distant from the medical staff, nurses, case managers, and revenue cycle colleagues. Some large hospital systems have centralized all UR activities and conduct virtual reviews for each acute care facility. At other hospitals, the UR specialists are on-site but are rarely seen on the patient care units. There are also hospitals where the UR specialists work from home with access to the EHR. In most of these models, email, electronic correspondence, and EHR apps create a link to alert the hospitalist of any documentation gaps. Although virtual models seem to work well for continuing-stay reviews, they are fundamentally less suited to UR activities focused on the front end of the revenue cycle, such as in the ED and providing real-time medical documentation coaching and admission decision guidance.

Each UR model has benefits and drawbacks. Whichever approach is used, maintaining an open line of communication between the UR specialists and the care team is critical to avoiding issues that could jeopardize revenue.

There are as many models of team meetings as there are hospitals, but daily structured multidisciplinary rounds focused on progression of care are a good way to enhance communication and collaboration between members of the care team in any given setting. A repeat of a nursing report should be avoided, and readers may want to consider the New England Medical Center model for rapid review of patients with emphasis on progression of care (throughput):

- *Plan for stay* – Remind everyone why the patient was admitted and what are the treatment plan goals.
- *Plan for the day* – What is the plan for today and can we expect any delays or obstacles?
- *Plan for the pay* – Are we doing anything that may put the patient or hospital at financial risk (e.g., excessive serial testing, nonformulary medications, indwelling catheter that should be removed, lengthy bed rest, diagnostics not relevant to reason for admission)?
- *Plan for the way* – What is the discharge plan? Have arrangements been made and are the patient and family prepared?

By focusing on these prompts, the team understands that it is working collaboratively to keep the patient's progression of care moving forward.

Morning hospitalist handoff rounds are often overlooked as an opportunity to share information. This is unfortunate, as they can be structured to be highly productive for the hospitalist, the UR specialist, and the care coordinator. We have attended many versions of morning handoff rounds and after the nocturnist gives their report, the lead hospitalist often "runs the list" to quickly review the status of each patient and attend to the issues that are raised by care team members. The advantage of having UR specialists attend these rounds is one of time: because the hospitalists rightfully prioritize their work, they may not make unit rounds and see the patient waiting for discharge or a follow-up procedure until later in the day.

Regardless of the format chosen, the first crucial step to creating multidisciplinary meetings is an executive commitment and willingness to address the situations that constrain teamwork. When this commitment comes from the top down, it makes a statement about the way that the hospital and health system do business. The way that the care team members interact affects quality outcomes. In fact, this human interaction is often missing, which leads to throughput and transition delays.

Role of the Physician Advisor

It is no longer a question of the value that a PA brings to the hospital, but rather a question of the scope of practice, whether one, two, or even three PAs are sufficient, or whether to consider a hybrid of a hospital-employed PA plus outsourced backup. The growth of this specialty is a direct result of the explosion of MA contracts, aggressive oversight auditors, constant debates over how to apply Medicare rules, and the volume of denials. It wasn't long ago that the role of PA was seen as a good pre-retirement option, a way to ease an experienced, well-respected physician out of clinical care and leverage their collegiality with their peers to influence documentation and discharge decisions. Today, the role is often filled by hospitalists who see it as an attractive adjunct to their clinical experience. Physicians in their early and midcareers may not want to take on a full-time PA role, but many express interest in expanding their responsibilities and participating in the business of health. In fact, Medscape's Young Physician Compensation Report 2020 states that 59% of physicians under the age of 40 are aiming for promotion (Medscape, 2020). Invariably, hospitalists see the chief medical officer (CMO) chair as a future goal and the role of the PA as a step up the ladder. Traditionally, internal medicine and family medicine provided a natural pathway to becoming a PA, but now physicians from less traditional specialties, such as pediatrics, surgical specialties, and radiology, are stepping into PA roles. In fact, the president of the American College of Physician Advisors at the time of this writing is a pediatric hospitalist.

A PA is considered part administrator and part physician and, depending upon the executive suite, may complement the role of the CMO, the vice president of medical affairs, or the CFO or may stand alone in the absence of those roles. Depending upon the size of the institution, the PA may provide advisory services for all the hospital's performance improvement initiatives or for specific programs such as quality, CDI, UR, or case management. In response to a 2019 ACMA survey, 44% of facilities reported that they had hospital-based PAs, while 32% had a combination of in-house and outsourced (American Case Management Association, 2019).

■ **Figure 4.3**

Sample physician advisor job description

Job summary:

The PA serves as a liaison between hospital administration, the department of case management, and the medical staff to address issues of resource and performance improvement. The PA reports case management data to the hospital performance improvement council and is a member of the hospital UR committee.

Essential duties:

- Serves as a resource to the case management team to advise them on how to best remedy a utilization issue
- Serves as a resource to the case management team to communicate with attending physicians, residents, and

Sample physician advisor job description (cont.)

other health professionals as needed in order to clarify issues regarding appropriateness of admission status and resource utilization, including criteria for continued stay in specialty units

- As requested by case managers, UR specialists, and/or counselors, reviews individual cases, including denied cases, to evaluate appropriateness of admission or continuing stay, applying professional judgment in the context of patient-specific variables

- Supports the case management department by reviewing and signing medical necessity appeal letters based on appropriateness of admission status and/or level of care

- Acts as spokesperson for care management activities in coordination with medical staff and hospital leadership

- Provides education and serves as a resource to medical staff colleagues regarding best practices, care management structures and functions, use of clinical guidelines, and alternative levels of care

- Analyzes utilization data and presents to medical staff individually and in meetings

- Participates in clinical process redesign and implementation (e.g., clinical pathway/algorithm development, preprinted order sheets, standing order sets, and clinical program development)

- Supports implementation of systemwide clinical initiatives, and participates in identification of opportunities and development and implementation of clinical practice standards for the healthcare system (process and content)

- Assists in identifying avoidable days and resource use opportunities and addresses these issues with individual physicians and/or practice leaders

- Coordinates and recommends communications for medical management initiatives

- Reviews resource utilization reports and performance measures to make recommendations to departments and the medical executive committee regarding opportunities for improvement in patient care, clinical documentation practices, resource utilization, and reduction of denials

- Provides input for design and implementation of automated information systems (e.g., order entry) to improve clinical care coordination

- Assists CDI specialists with physician communication and education relative to clinical documentation practices

- Interacts with governmental and commercial payers as required to clarify and address policies and procedures

Qualifications

- Licensed physician with a minimum of five years' clinical practice experience

- Active member of the healthcare system medical staff and participating member of various medical committees

- Strong clinical judgment and technical ability

- Understands alternative reimbursement options and general contract terms

- Well-demonstrated skills with case review/case management

- Strong collaboration skills with other physicians

- Knowledgeable in utilization management and basic principles of quality assessment

- Excellent interpersonal and communication skills

- Availability and willingness to complete educational opportunities related to the position

Source: Ronald Hirsch, MD, FACP, CHCQM, CHRI, vice president, R1 Physician Advisory Services in Chicago. Reprinted with permission.

Physicians are increasingly burnt out by the environment and the sense that how they do their jobs is always questioned. This may make them disinclined to participate in improvement activities. However, physician participation in efforts to improve the value of care is essential. Physicians control most testing and treatment decisions, and their documentation is the foundation on which nearly all revenue cycle processes are based. Programs to improve documentation, status decisions, and transitions of care will be less likely to succeed if physicians aren't fully on board. Despite all the communication efforts put forth by the executive team to engage the medical staff in the business of managing care, it is perhaps the PA who is best positioned to bridge the gap. Though the C-suite may have a medical executive, it is the PA who possesses the practical information and regulatory expertise that physicians need to successfully wade through today's hospital environment.

The PA is prepared to understand and interpret the myriad of payer regulations that dictate what qualifies as patient status, inpatient or outpatient, and level of care for claims reimbursement and what payers consider to be medically necessary and, therefore, covered services. They must try to maximize compliant revenue and combat potential claim denials over status and continuing-stay decisions. And they must be able to promote hospital-physician alignment. Even with ongoing hospital acquisitions of physician practices, employment does not equal cooperation, and the PA is in a better position to forge cooperation and establish a rapport than an administrator without clinical experience.

PAs serve as liaisons between clinical staff, payers, and administrative personnel. They help the organization and the medical staff navigate the intricacies of Medicare regulations, contractual obligations, and payment rules and offer valuable guidance to determine medical necessity of care, assess resource utilization, champion compliance, and improve clinical documentation processes. They look at cases with the eye of a UR specialist or a payer's medical director, which is a perspective most practicing physicians don't have.

The PA serves as an essential resource for the UR specialist in medical necessity determinations.

Admission medical necessity is a two-step process. The UR specialist first applies screening criteria that serves as a guide for further exploration and then considers the patient's clinical presentation as documented by the physician. When the patient's condition as documented by the physician does not meet or exceed inpatient admission screening criteria but the physician feels strongly that the patient should be admitted as an inpatient, Medicare permits a physician to apply "complex medical judgment." In the face of ambiguous clinical documentation, the UR specialist will seek more information from the physician and may suggest the physician include additional documentation to better reflect that "complex medical judgment." However, if secondary review is required, the expertise of the PA is invaluable. The PA will assess the entire case and may recommend, based on the physician's documentation of the clinical situation, inpatient hospital level of care even when national criteria aren't met or they may recommend that the patient be placed in outpatient/observation.

Depending upon the size of the hospital and the number of PAs, it is not uncommon for the PA to maintain a small practice presence; in fact, doing so often contributes to the PA's credibility among peers. Some PAs remain as members of a small-group private practice or provide care in a hospital-owned clinic. However, the nature of such practice depends heavily on the hospital's size, the volume of cases normally requiring review, and the additional duties assigned to the PA. It is not in the hospital's interest to allow the PA to practice as a hospitalist, as doing so would cast the PA as a competitor with the private physicians who continue to admit their own patients. Likewise, it is difficult for a practicing specialist to serve as PA because he or she may have difficulty providing feedback to a physician on whom he or she depends for referrals. As a member of the UR committee or, more often, chairperson, the PA is often called upon to review admissions for changes to outpatient using the condition code 44 process. If the PA is providing any care to that patient, then the PA would be unable to participate in that process and another physician member of the UR committee would have to replace the PA, creating a delay.

The following caveat about the relationship between the PA and the UR specialist is expressed in *The Leader's Guide to Hospital Case Management* and has withstood the test of time:

> With the exception of serious quality-of-care situations—and in those cases, the risk manager should also be involved—the [PA] should not ride shotgun to the driver of the stagecoach. There is no better way to undermine the [UR specialist's] efforts to build a relationship with her [physician] partner than to bring in a physician to speak for her. Rather, the [physician] advisor, who "walks in the skin" of the attending physician, can help the [UR specialist] distance herself emotionally from the situation and objectively review the options open to her. (Ramey and Daniels, 2005)

Scope of PA responsibilities

There is no standard amount of time that a PA will spend working in an advisory role, although the 2019 ACMA survey reports that 41% of hospitals have the benefit of a full-time PA. The presence of a full-time PA expands the scope of the PA's role and generally encompasses UR and CDI support, denials/appeals, resource utilization, compliance, quality, and chairmanship of the UR committee. Erik DeLue, MD, the medical director of Virtua Voorhees in New Jersey and the director of physician utilization review for the entire Virtua system, says that as a rule of thumb, he hires one PA to support every 15 or 20 hospitalists (Maguire, 2018).

Another variable is the percentage of community physicians who tend to be more conservative and averse to engaging in conversations they may perceive as challenging their autonomy. The practical reality is that, with some rare exceptions, community physicians respond better to peer-to-peer suggestions than they do to suggestions from an administrative representative.

Given the growth of regulatory, payment, coding, compliance, quality, and documentation issues, it is advisable to have a physician on staff who is invested in the business of managing care. Hospitals with an average daily census (ADC) of less than 300 should have one full-time PA, with the exception of CAHs and small community hospitals with an ADC of fewer than 100, which are often best suited for contracted resources. A full-time PA generally has seven major role responsibilities:

1. Advisory: The PA is generally the primary resource to the UR specialists, the CDI team, and the case managers to help them create the best plan of action to overcome obstacles that affect patient flow, resource utilization, and discharge.

2. Administration: Case review for determination of the proper admission status makes up the bulk of the administrative duties of the PA. The advisor reviews specific cases and interacts directly with the treating physician or the payer's medical director to mediate differences and negotiate resolution.

3. Education: The PA serves as a subject matter expert to proactively consult with the treating physicians and the patient's care team regarding the appropriate utilization of acute care resources and essential documentation. The educational opportunities can be informal one-on-one conversations on the patient care units, or they can be held in more formal venues, such as committee meetings or patient care conferences.

4. Orientation: The PA provides onboarding education to medical students, interns, and residents to acquaint each with the realities of the business of healthcare and how the PA will interact with them on matters relating to documentation, medical necessity status assignment, and regulatory requirements.

5. Medical staff liaison: The PA is the conduit of information to the medical staff, the executive team, and the board of trustees on issues pertaining to the federal or state regulatory environment, payer issues, and resource utilization successes and challenges. As liaison, the PA does the following:

   – Interprets federal and state regulations' impact on medical practice

   – Advises the medical community of new or revised rules that affect practice

   – Consults on resource utilization issues

   – Promotes communication and exchange of best practice information

   – Markets the value of the role of the UR specialist to the medical community

   – Collaborates with individual physicians to improve utilization outcomes

6. Policy development: As regulations change, so do expectations. The PA collaborates with compliance officers and legal resources to develop policies and processes to support new programs or changing regulatory and accrediting agency requirements.

7. Advocacy: As a member or chairperson of the UR committee, the PA advocates high-quality, cost-effective care for hospitalized patients and collaborates with colleagues and the decision support team to identify opportunities to improve performance outcomes based on outcome metrics.

Hospitals with an ADC of greater than 300 may want to consider having two physicians serving as advisors. The first PA would serve as the internal consultant to the medical staff. This PA is often seen in larger community or teaching facilities and routinely travels through the patient care units looking for opportunities to network and consult with treating physicians. He or she offers real-time, point-of-care coaching and information on documentation, use of protocols, resource management initiatives, and up-to-date information on regulatory or contractual issues. This PA meets regularly with key medical staff champions to explore opportunities to improve practice performance and offers one-on-one counseling when warranted. The second PA would be positioned as the primary liaison between the treating physician and the payer to contest concurrent denials and work the appeal process with his or her commercial payer counterparts or the Recovery Audit Contractor, MAC, or administrative law judge representatives in the case of recoupment efforts. There are also models where the work responsibilities of the PA are dependent upon the payer. One PA becomes the Medicare expert and knowledgeable about the rules and regs governing management of original Medicare patients, while the other PA serves as the resource for commercial payers and is current on contractual obligations and participates in all contract language negotiations.

C-suite leaders are rarely cognizant of the depth of PA involvement and management of the UR activities on a day-to-day basis. They tend to assume that assigning specific PA responsibilities to a group of loyal community physicians and/or hospitalists will suffice. However, in our experience, a part-time, informal presence falls short of expectations. A dedicated PA is expected to serve as a consultant and resource to every physician regarding hospitalization appropriateness, inpatient or observation status, resource utilization, regulatory requirements, and length-of-stay management and will serve as liaison to coding, documentation specialists, medical records, and third-party payers when necessary. According to a conversation we had with John Zelem, MD, a practicing PA, medical peers and colleagues may offer opinions on documentation and regulatory interpretations, but with expert knowledge of the business of managing care, the PA is best positioned to offer informed recommendations.

The PA and the new marketplace

The PA's role is changing as hospitals enter into shared savings or accountable care organizations. Because many of these arrangements involve the full continuum of care and some form of shared savings based on financial and quality outcomes, the PA is often best positioned to offer insights and advice about how to streamline service delivery, use and apply evidence-based protocols across the continuum, and serve as advisor to practices offering chronic care and transitional care services. The value of the PA cannot be overstated.

Several organizations offer certification for UR- and UM-related activities that may be of interest to PAs. The primary agency offering such certification is the ABQAURP. It offers a core body of knowledge to fulfill the educational requirements for sitting for the Physician Advisor Sub-Specialty of Health Care Quality and Management (HCQM) certifying exam.

In 2013, the American College of Physician Advisors (ACPA) was formed, and it is now recognized as the professional organization for PAs. The ACPA blog, newsletter, and member forums provide up-to-date information relevant to the PA scope of practice as well as educational and networking opportunities.

The Healthcare Finance Management Association (HFMA) offers certification as a revenue cycle representative (CRCR). The CRCR certification applies primarily to personnel directly and indirectly associated with the revenue cycle, such as UR specialists, compliance managers, PAs, and managed care contract coordinators.

In addition to the ACPA and the ABQAURP, there are several external physician advisory service organizations, such as R1™ Physician Advisory Solutions and Sound Physicians Advisory Services, each of which also provide well-respected training programs to keep PAs current on regulatory issues and best practices.

Each PA must be able to demonstrate a return on investment (ROI) that warrants their salary. The executive sponsor must establish objectives that link to compensation incentives for each employment contract cycle. The more effective the PA is in influencing the use of evidence-based practice, reducing inappropriate resource utilization, or reducing or overturning denials, the greater the PA's compensation. Make the most of this powerful incentive, but be careful not to overincentivize. Because the PA's work often reduces the utilization of services, the structure of any compensation incentive must comply with laws concerning shared savings so that it does not appear that the PA is paid to deny care to patients.

Outsourced resources

Commercial PA services are popular but often costly. In general, these remote physicians have the opportunity to review the documentation confirming medical necessity through dedicated portals and/or a conversation with the UR specialist before making direct, peer-to-peer contact with the attending physician to discuss the issues and reach a successful resolution. While some hospitals employ only internal PAs for a limited number of hours, the outsourced PAs are available whenever needed. They will also represent the hospital and attending physician in peer-to-peer conversations with payers to defend the chosen status. This allows the internal PA to concentrate on other activities and allows the practicing physicians to do what they do best, which is take care of patients.

Today, a combination of a first- and second-level review may be essential to promote full compliance with the *CoP*, the expectations of the oversight agencies, and the requirements of the commercial insurance companies. Failure to review cases as part of a front-end revenue cycle program may result in a complex and fragmented system of back-end rework that will hinder the organization's ability to reduce the risk of payer denials, the recoupment of payments, and the scrutiny of the oversight agencies. The organization will also incur avoidable costs and revenue stream delays.

Ethical Obligations for Utilization Review

The origin of medical ethics traces back to the Hippocratic Oath, which was written during the Classical Greek period. The oath, which appears in Figure 4.4, has been modified through the years as references to the gods of Ancient Greece were removed and modifications were made to reflect modern medical practice. The most commonly used version was written in 1964 by Dr. Louis Lasagna, academic dean of the School of Medicine at Tufts University in Medford, Massachusetts.

■ **Figure 4.4**

The Hippocratic Oath
I swear to fulfill, to the best of my ability and judgment, this covenant:
I will respect the hard-won scientific gains of those physicians in whose steps I walk, and gladly share such knowledge as is mine with those who are to follow.
I will apply, for the benefit of the sick, all measures which are required, avoiding those twin traps of over-treatment and therapeutic nihilism.
I will remember that there is art to medicine as well as science, and that warmth, sympathy, and understanding may outweigh the surgeon's knife or the chemist's drug.
I will not be ashamed to say "I know not," nor will I fail to call in my colleagues when the skills of another are needed for a patient's recovery.
I will respect the privacy of my patients, for their problems are not disclosed to me that the world may know. Most especially must I tread with care in matters of life and death. If it is given me to save a life, all thanks. But it may also be within my power to take a life; this awesome responsibility must be faced with great humbleness and awareness of my own frailty. Above all, I must not play at God.
I will remember that I do not treat a fever chart, a cancerous growth, but a sick human being, whose illness may affect the person's family and economic stability. My responsibility includes these related problems, if I am to care adequately for the sick.
I will prevent disease whenever I can, for prevention is preferable to cure.
I will remember that I remain a member of society, with special obligations to all my fellow human beings, those sound of mind and body, as well as the infirm.
If I do not violate this oath, may I enjoy life and art, respected while I live and remembered with affection hereafter. May I always act so as to preserve the finest traditions of my calling and may I long experience the joy of healing those who seek my help.

There are also codes of ethics produced by professional societies, such as the American Medical Association and the American Nurses Association, and most hospitals have a multidisciplinary ethics committee.

Principles of medical ethics

The four basic principles of medical ethics are autonomy, beneficence, nonmaleficence, and justice.

Autonomy

Autonomy refers to a patient's right to control what happens to his or her body. In most cases, this refers to a patient's right to refuse a treatment that the care team recommends. The patient's care team has a duty to ensure that the patient and family are fully informed about the procedure's risks and benefits, including the costs and coverage by the payer. On the surface, it seems that cost and coverage should not be a consideration in a patient's decision to accept or reject a recommended treatment. However, for patients without health insurance or those who have health insurance with a high deductible or copayment, concern about the cost of care may equal or exceed the concern about the medical condition itself. Though researchers disagree on the evidence for medical bills causing bankruptcies, a 2017 Consumer Report noted that although medical bankruptcies have declined since the passage of the Affordable Care Act (ACA) in 2010, from a high of 1,536,7990 filings that year to 770,846 filings in 2016, medical costs remain a serious concern for many Americans (St. John, 2017). In 2020, Gallup reported more than a fifth of American adults skipped a test or a medical treatment that their physician recommended because it was too expensive (Saad, 2019). Many attribute the physician epidemic of overtesting to the fee-for-service payment structure and litigious environment in the United States, leading many patients to question whether they really need the tests that their physicians order.

Discussions about fee-for-service have centered on the fact that many medical tests and procedures are ordered to rule out a medical condition and are not likely to actually identify the condition. For example, a doctor may order an MRI for a patient with back pain to rule out an epidural abscess or other serious cause. It is perfectly reasonable for a patient to inquire as to the doctor's impression of the risk for such conditions (e.g., there may be a 1% chance of finding the condition) and the risk of not discovering such a condition in a timely manner (e.g., paralysis if an epidural abscess is present and not discovered). Physicians should also inform patients about the risks of the procedure itself—including the risk of any radiation or intravenous contrast required—and the test's accuracy. The patient can use that information to make an informed decision about whether to undergo the procedure or whether to accept the risk of not receiving a diagnosis in a timely manner. In many cases, the physician will request that the patient sign a form indicating that he or she is declining treatment against medical advice (AMA). Signing an AMA form does not mean that the patient can no longer be treated by the physician or the facility; it only acknowledges that the patient has made an informed decision to decline that specific test or procedure, and other types of evaluation and treatment can proceed as necessary. It should be noted that the signed AMA form does not in itself absolve the physician from all responsibility, nor does the absence of a signed form mean the physician is de facto negligent. Rather, it is the content of the conversation between the patient and the physician, and documentation of that conversation, that will determine if the patient truly made an informed choice.

The use of evidence-based shared decision-making tools is rapidly expanding as a way to help promote patient autonomy and reduce tension between the patient and provider. In fact, CMS requires using an evidence-based shared decision-making tool within the national coverage determination (NCD) for implanted cardioverter defibrillators, which are being considered for use in patients for primary prevention of life-threatening arrhythmias. CMS also requires using a shared decision-making tool on anticoagulation treatments before placing a left atrial appendage occlusion device.

Patients who wish to decline tests because of cost alone should be required to consult with the patient financial services staff to attempt to arrange a payment plan or find alternative payment sources, such as a charity fund. Discussions about the patient's ability to pay for care should not take place with patients in the emergency department until they have undergone a medical screening examination and stabilization, as required by the Emergency Medical Treatment and Active Labor Act (EMTALA).

Decision-making capability

The care team must ensure that a patient who is refusing treatment is properly informed and capable of making such a decision. Contrary to common belief, this is not a determination of competence, which is a legal concept—rather, a treating practitioner must determine a patient's decision-making capacity. Despite what happens in hospitals around the country, decision-making capacity can be determined by any treating practitioner, not just a psychiatrist who is trained to diagnose and treat psychiatric illness. Decision-making capacity can change over time—even over the course of a single day. The key is to remember that the process of determining decision-making capacity is about the patient's decision-making *process*, independent of the patient's final treatment decision. (See Figure 4.5.)

■ Figure 4.5

Criteria for decision-making capacity

1. Ability to express a choice: "Can you tell me what your decision is?"

2. Ability to understand the relevant information: "Please tell me, in your own words, what you know and understand about:

   - Your condition

   - The treatment being recommended

   - The risks and benefits of the treatment

   - Any other options that have been discussed (including no treatment)

   - The (outcomes and consequences) risks and benefits of those options (including no treatment)"

3. Ability to appreciate one's situation:

   - "Can you tell me what you believe is wrong with you?"

   - "Do you believe that you need treatment?"

   - "Do you understand what will happen if you do not have treatment?"

4. Ability to reason with the relevant information:

   - "Would you share with me how you reached your decision?"

   - "What factors did you consider when making your decision?"

Source: Applebaum, P. (2007, November 1). Assessment of Patients' Competence to Consent to Treatment. New England Journal of Medicine. https://www. nejm.org/doi/full/10.1056/NEJMcp074045.

If a provider does not believe that a patient has decision-making capacity, then a surrogate decision-maker must be consulted. Each hospital should have a policy on appointing a surrogate decision-maker based on state and federal law and the durable power of attorney for healthcare, if available. Provide the surrogate decision-maker with the patient's advance directives and any other indications of the patient's previously stated wishes about healthcare, such as the patient's completed Physician Orders for Life-Sustaining

Treatment. The UR specialist is often involved in this process as an intermediary between the care team, the patient, and the payer, and he or she may be called upon to explore other options for care, including transfer to a provider or institution that will honor the patient's expressed healthcare decisions if they cannot be met at the current hospital.

Beneficence

Beneficence refers to the provider's obligation to do what is right for the patient's health and well-being. A UR specialist demonstrates beneficence by advocating for a patient to receive the care required to treat his or her condition. In an attempt to limit costs, some payers seek to limit advanced post-hospital care by refusing to approve a transfer to acute rehabilitation, a long-term acute care hospital, a skilled nursing facility (SNF), or home health services. The UR specialist should be aware of common criteria for use of such post-hospital services and ensure that the payer has the necessary information to approve the service within the patient's benefit.

As an expert in utilization criteria, the UR specialist might also note that a patient is not receiving care that appears to be indicated for the patient's condition. For example, he or she may note that a patient who is ready for discharge and appears to demonstrate a need for home health services has no home health ordered. The UR specialist should discuss such a situation with the patient's nurse or case manager and offer to make the appropriate referrals. The busy environment of the hospital often interferes with providing personalized care to patients, but while a UR specialist's job description does not typically include finding appropriate candidates for home care, based on the concept of beneficence, spending a few extra moments to do so may have a profound effect on the patient's future—and may help avoid a readmission.

Nonmaleficence

The most obvious ethical concept, **nonmaleficence** ("do no harm"), is often the most difficult to balance. No treatment is free from potential harm. For example, a patient having a simple blood test may incur a financial cost that could be considered a harm. The patient may develop bleeding from a venipuncture or get a superficial infection at the site. A test may reveal an incidental abnormality that requires more invasive testing, or the test result could be erroneously abnormal and lead to further testing. The patient also may acquire iatrogenic anemia due to questionable serial blood lab tests. Likewise, many tests are done to rule out a rare disease, but in doing so, they subject the patient to real risks, including exposure to radiation, development of an allergic reaction, or kidney injury from intravenous dye. Such tests may have incidental results that require further evaluation. Thus, the benefits and risks of every intervention must be weighed.

Even commonly accepted screening tests—including a screening mammography for women and prostate-specific antigen testing for men—may cause harm. The National Cancer Institute estimates that if 10,000 women have a mammogram at age 60, up to 50 cancer deaths will be averted, but almost 1,000 women will have a false positive mammogram that requires a potentially disfiguring biopsy. Nearly 50,000 women in the United States each year are diagnosed and treated for ductal carcinoma in situ, a condition of abnormal cells inside a milk duct in the breast. The cells are noninvasive and cannot spread outside the breast, although treatment is recommended if the mass of abnormal cells becomes large. However, doctors don't know how to differentiate between cases that will develop an invasive cancer and those that won't (McCarthy, 2017).

The most common nonmaleficence role for the UR specialist may be when a physician orders a test or procedure that the patient's payer does not cover. Such a situation could arise for many reasons. For example, the patient may have a high-deductible plan or may have a limited coverage plan, although this situation happens less frequently now due to the minimum coverage requirements of the ACA. Often, the patient's clinical situation does not match the payer's coverage policies. In that case, the UR specialist should obtain a copy of the coverage decision and coverage policy and review the case with the ordering physician or refer the situation to the patient's nurse or case manager. The UR specialist can work with the team to determine whether additional information can be conveyed to the payer, whether another procedure or test can be substituted, or whether the patient actually needs the ordered test or procedure.

Although we always want to believe that physicians are acting in the patient's best interest, this is not always the case. There may be times when the physician has not kept up with advances in medical care and orders a test or procedure that will not benefit the patient. Unfortunately, there are also rare situations in which the physician may order a test or perform a procedure purely for his or her personal financial gain. If such situations arise, the UR specialist should immediately confer with the patient's nurse or case manager to try to resolve the issue at the point of care with the physician. If that fails, refer the case to the PA or notify the UR supervisor so that it can be properly investigated.

Justice

Justice requires providers to be as fair as possible when offering treatments and allocating scarce resources. This ethical concept may be the most difficult to adopt in clinical practice, as it requires balancing the good of the individual patient with the good of society. Healthcare in the United States is largely government funded, whether it be through Medicare, Medicaid, the Veterans Administration, Tricare (for active military and families), or subsidies under the ACA. United States healthcare spending grew 4.6% in 2019, reaching $3.8 trillion or $11,582 per person. Health spending accounted for 17.7% of the gross domestic product in 2019 (CMS, 2020). Most Americans are opposed to increasing taxes to pay for this increase, which means that every tax dollar spent on healthcare is a dollar that is not available for other expenses, such as repairing the country's aging infrastructure or educating the country's children. The UR specialist—or any individual provider, for that matter—cannot tell a patient that a needed service is not available because the money is being spent patching the potholes on the city's streets or providing all-day kindergarten for children.

However, many of the healthcare services provided to patients are not truly medically necessary or have little chance of improving the patient's health and well-being. In a survey report published in 2017, physicians reported that 20.6% of overall medical care was unnecessary, including 22.0% of prescription medications, 24.9% of tests, and 11.1% of procedures (Lyu, 2017). A ProPublica article in 2018 confirmed these findings and reported that an estimated $765 billion a year is spent on unnecessary tests, procedures, and hospitalizations (Allen, 2018).

Furthermore, many interventions are provided to patients without shared decision-making—that is, a thoughtful discussion between the patient and the provider about the risks of, benefits of, and alternatives to a treatment. This is most evident in the ICU, where expensive, invasive, and painful technology is often used not to keep people alive but rather to prolong their dying process. Much of this care is provided without asking the patient or decision-maker what he or she really wants. Of course, this discussion is best held when an immediate decision is not necessary, prior to admission to the ICU. Best-selling author and practicing surgeon Atul Gawande discusses this issue in his book, *Being Mortal,* when he writes that "scientific advances have turned the processes of aging and dying into medical experiences, matters to be managed by healthcare professionals. And we in the medical world have proved alarmingly unprepared for it."

Justice also plays a role in the review of payment for health services by payers. This ethical principle requires that payers reviewing coverage decisions for patients make their decisions based on the established policies of medical necessity and published guidelines. Payers should not base their decisions on a structure that rewards the reviewer for denying payment. The appeal processes should be fair and not influenced by financial considerations. Some would say that the current Recovery Audit program started by CMS in 2009 is not just, as the contractors are paid based on a contingency fee, which essentially means that they are paid for denying claims.

The UR specialist must uphold these four ethical concepts when interacting with patients, providers, and payers. In the United States, access to medical services is not an absolute right—and patients cannot dictate what services physicians and other providers must deliver, while payers are not obligated to pay for care that is not covered or determined to be not necessary. Therefore, providers should not withhold care based solely on the ability to pay.

Legal Considerations

Regulatory compliance

The most important legal precept for the UR specialist is to not break the law. Chapter 2 reviews all the regulatory bodies and policies pertinent to the UR specialist's work. Because payments made to hospitals and providers for regular Medicare and Medicaid patients come from a federal agency, fraudulent activity will be prosecuted as a federal crime. The federal government takes improper payments seriously. For example, CMS estimated in 2020 that the Medicare fee-for-service (FFS) improper payment rate was 6.27% (approximately $25.7 billion) and the Medicaid improper payment rate was 21.36% (approximately $86.49 billion), while the Part C, or MA, rate was 6.78% or approximately $16.27 billion (CMS, November 2020). "Improper payments" include overpayments as well as fraudulent claims. Before the UR specialist starts worrying about prosecution for Medicare fraud, though, know that the federal government notes that although all fraud is improper, the majority of improper payments are due to payment errors, not fraud. The federal government describes three categories of payment errors, one of which is medical necessity errors—an area where the UR specialist has great influence.

Also consider the source of information. The advent of the internet and social media has made it easy for personal opinions and interpretations to be widely disseminated without any independent verification or vetting. For example, when the 2-midnight rule was implemented in October 2013, widespread confusion about the rule led CMS to announce a delay in audits and rule enforcement. But several organizations incorrectly reported that CMS had delayed implementation (rather than enforcement) of the rule, leading many to believe that admission decisions should continue to be made with the prior guidance based on risk. The removal of surgeries from the inpatient-only list has led some to state that as a result all such surgeries must be performed as outpatient. That is clearly not correct.

Medicare Administrative Contractors (MAC) interpret Medicare regulations and give education to providers. Because the regulations are promulgated by CMS, remember that answers from a MAC representative show his or her interpretation of the Medicare regulation, but the source of truth is CMS itself. As with CMS, MAC education is provided via written materials, teleconferences, webinars, and Web-based educational tools. When seeking answers to regulatory questions, if you find that CMS guidance is not sufficient, the first alternative to turn to should be the MACs.

As an example of this process, on 15 February 2018, CMS released a decision memorandum to update the NCD for coverage of implanted cardioverter defibrillators. One of the changes removed the requirement to report all patient data to a national registry before submitting a claim. In the past, to confirm this requirement, the provider was required to place modifier -Q0 on the claim to notify the MAC that the NCD requirements were met. And in fact, the MACs had an automatic edit that rejected a claim without modifier -Q0. However, CMS failed to issue a timely new payment instruction to the MACs, which continued to reject claims without modifier -Q0 even though it was no longer required.

One way to monitor regulatory compliance is through audits. All claims for any medical service, whether for a patient covered by a federally funded insurance program or one covered by a commercial plan, are subject to audit. In September 2012, CMS started having contractors in selected states perform prepayment audits, where the clinical information is reviewed prior to the claim being paid. This reduces "pay and chase," as the claim is not paid until the information is verified. This tactic has drastically reduced the amount of home care and durable medical equipment fraud, as it was common for providers of those services with criminal intent to obtain a Medicare provider number, bill a large number of fraudulent claims, and then close up shop and disappear once the claims were paid. The prepayment review demonstration took place in just 11 states, during which time RACs prevented $192.8 million in improper payments from leaving the program. The demonstration was intended as a three-year project but was paused and never reinstated.

Nevertheless, the value of audits is not disputed, and many hospitals do their own audits using key indicators as a trigger to hold the claim until the case is reviewed. Some hospitals use the dollar amount of the claim as an indicator, while others will pull certain diagnoses, such as chest pain. In larger hospitals, the compliance department often lead the effort for internal audit. This department may publish a schedule that is distributed to department heads who are encouraged to do their own internal audit using small samples of target areas.

With all these retrospective audits of claims—whether pre- or post-payment—the insurer or contractor hired to perform the audit will review the clinical information provided at the time of authorization and claim submission and compare it to the clinical information documented in the medical record. If the medical record does not support the medical necessity of the service, the claim will be denied. This emphasizes the value of an internal audit process targeted at high-risk cases to double-check all the parameters that may put the claim at risk.

The OIG has been performing audits of hospitals for many years but only recently began to extrapolate their findings. For example, if a hospital submits 100 claims for a service, the OIG will audit 10 claims. If four of the 10 are found to be improper, the OIG will extrapolate from that finding and ask for a refund for 40 of the 100 claims. The use of extrapolation exponentially increases the financial risk of audits to hospitals and makes compliance with all rules and regulations more important than ever.

The OIG is also not shy about recommending criminal charges against providers who commit fraud. One notorious case involved the now defunct Forest Park Medical Center, a physician-owned surgical hospital, which was accused of paying and receiving bribes and kickbacks of approximately $40 million in exchange for referrals of Medicare and Medicaid patients as well as patients with out-of-network private insurance. In this case, the Department of Justice also evoked the 1961 Travel Act by accusing the hospital of unlawful activities using facilities of interstate commerce to induce potential out-of-network patients by paying for travel and lodging (Department of Justice, March 2021).

The DOJ also collects financial penalties from organizations that are in violation of the law. In 2020, the DOJ recovered $2.2 billion in false claims from the healthcare industry (Department of Justice, January 2021).

Patients seeking insurance coverage for benefits to which they are not entitled may also attempt to encourage providers to give false information. For example, a Medicare patient may ask to be admitted as an inpatient and kept in the hospital for three days in order to access his or her Part A SNF benefit. Whether minor or major, all instances of misrepresentation by providers or patients are fraudulent, as they are intentional actions taken to obtain some benefit or advantage to which the patient is not otherwise entitled. The UR specialist should not take part in any fraudulent behavior and should consult with the hospital compliance officer if there is any suggestion of fraud.

Asking the compliance officer to review a situation does not mean that the UR specialist is accusing the physician or patient of fraud; it is merely seeking clarity by having the person whose job it is to have deep regulatory knowledge and understanding of healthcare compliance review the situation. UR specialists should not fear retribution for asking for such an opinion; there should be an environment within the hospital where compliance is everyone's job.

The hospital must self-disclose improper payments of any kind when they are discovered. The OIG has established a 60-day rule for such self-disclosure of improper payments. If a hospital self-discloses and returns any improper payments it may have received within 60 days of discovery, then the hospital will not be subject to the onerous penalties of the False Claims Act, which include a $10,000-per-day financial penalty and possible exclusion from the Medicare and Medicaid programs. Ideally, a well-organized hospital's chief compliance officer will find the improper payments and start that 60-day clock. However, if fraud is suspected by a UR specialist or any hospital staff, time is of the essence in reporting it.

Regulatory guidance

When seeking guidance on how to interpret a Medicare regulation, look not only at the source of the information but also at the information's validity. The federal government has a clear hierarchy for guidance. The Medicare statute is at the top as the ultimate regulatory authority, followed by regulations issued by CMS within the *Code of Federal Regulations* (*CFR*). Title 42 of the *CFR* encompasses regulations related to public health, and CMS develops manuals from these regulations to help providers and contractors interpret them, including:

- The *Medicare Benefit Policy Manual* is a 16-chapter guide to CMS' program issuances and day-to-day operating instructions, policies, and procedures that are based on CMS statutes, regulations, guidelines, models, and directives. The chapters each address a different area of coverage, from inpatient hospital services to SNF services to medical devices.

- *Medicare Claims Processing Manual* includes billing requirements and instructions across the spectrum of covered Medicare services and also includes appeal instructions and patient liability guidance.

In addition, CMS also releases informational documents, such as frequently asked questions or fact sheets, and holds open-door forum calls and webinars to provide other learning opportunities for healthcare workers. The MACs also educate providers on regulations and produce their own written publications, as well as educational teleconferences and webinars. As with CMS, all MACs have email lists for which people can sign up to receive notifications about all new publications and events.

HIPAA

The daily work of the UR specialist also requires adherence to the Health Insurance Portability and Accountability Act of 1996 (HIPAA), which protects the confidentiality and security of patients' protected health information (PHI). The UR specialist must be wary about becoming a HIPAA zealot and should remember that the "P" in HIPAA does not stand for privacy. We have encountered situations where fear of reprisal and lack of training leads to UR specialists misinterpreting or misapplying the law. Note that HIPAA specifically permits hospital staff to use or disclose PHI—without the individual's authorization—to a spouse, family members, friends, or other persons or parties identified by a patient for the purpose of treatment, payment, and healthcare operations activities. The rule was never intended to prevent providers from sharing information with others involved with care, nor was its purpose to prevent family members, others identified by the patient, and patients themselves from obtaining information. Still, it is important that the UR specialist confirms the identity of the person or entity requesting the information and that the information is used for one of the permitted activities.

Training and Education

Training

While the health sector has typically been insulated from job loss during periods of economic recession, the economic downturn of 2020–2021 is unique in that it is driven by a pandemic. As a result, healthcare revenue fell sharply in 2020, and more than 1.5 million healthcare jobs were lost. Hospitals are slowly recovering, but the applicant pool is small. Over the years, hospitals have shrunk their education and training budgets and have stripped workforce development opportunities. Others are entrenched in legacy programs that have damaged employee morale and left staff unprepared for market changes. According to feedback we've received from human resource directors, lack of career development is the number one reason millennials and GenXers, who make up about half of the hospital workforce, leave. Hospitals cannot afford to continue to shrink education and training budgets. The Association for Talent Development reports that healthcare organizations spend half on training programs compared to other industries and about a third less hours compared to the average of 34.1 hours for other industries (Modern Healthcare, 2019). To attract and retain an energized and loyal workforce, healthcare organizations are turning to more substantial onboarding and continuous training programs to attract candidates, retain current talent, and extend the knowledge of healthcare business to all hospital associates.

It's no longer acceptable to deny the financial burden many hospitalizations place on patients, and the entire care team must give consideration to the long-term financial repercussions of their care and service decisions. With proper training, the UR specialist will learn how to advocate for the patient and may offer less costly but equally effective alternatives to the physician as opposed to hospitalization. With proper training, the UR specialist will learn how to promote the use of evidence-based protocols to conserve resources and prevent avoidable interventions that are unwarranted. With proper training, the UR specialist will be able to identify opportunities to obtain benefits for un- or underinsured patients. The *American Journal of Medicine* reported that nearly half of people who experience medical bankruptcy named hospital bills as their biggest expense (Himmelstein, 2009). And in 2018, hospital bad debt across the country totaled $56.5 billion (Shoemaker, 2019).

There are two paths to take when training a successful UR specialist. One path, and the one most often encountered, takes the new team member through the required hospital orientation and regulatory-mandated courses and then partners the new recruit with a seasoned team member to serve as a mentor for the new team member and teach him or her the daily routine of task completion. Along the way, the mentor will introduce the new team member to the criteria used in the department, how to use various software applications, how to review charts, how to share information with the business office, and the best way to get in touch with the nurse, case manager, PA, and/or hospitalists using text, email, or phone calls. The mentoring period typically lasts between two and four weeks. In our opinion, this traditional approach devalues the critical importance of the UR specialist and often deprives the newcomer of the latest regulatory and contractual information needed to become an expert in their field. Passing along old information, misinformation, assumptions, and rumors from one generation of UR specialists to the next generation is not in the best interest of the profession nor the organization. The new recruit may pick up questionable practices that have been handed down from one generation of UR specialists to another without really understanding the reasons behind the practice or whether it is necessary. One UR specialist once told us that Medicare requires every patient chart to be reviewed every three days to make sure that it meets criteria. Although there is no such regulation, that's what he was told during his orientation, and that's what he is bound to pass on to the next recruit.

The value of onboarding

Industry-leading healthcare organizations don't limit training to the required courses, nor do they rely solely on mentoring to educate new staff members. Thus, the second path of training leads the new recruit through a comprehensive onboarding process that begins with a classroom program on the goals and purpose of the revenue cycle in general and the UR program specifically and how they support the hospital's mission. The classroom program uses presentations, case studies, and guest speakers as part of a formal development program that includes different levels of training over time. It is of even greater importance to expose young physicians, medical students, and residents to the business of healthcare because it impacts the decisions they will be making on behalf of their patients. In our experience, newcomers to the hospital environment appreciate any new information on how hospitals work and the issues affecting its success and, by association, their employment. Perhaps that's the impetus for the recent explosion of the "state of the hospital" conversations that execs are regularly holding with hospital associates of every variety. We have attended several of these assemblies and can report that they are very well attended and typically invite feedback by ending the session with the question "What can we do today to reduce risk and improve the quality of care for our patients?"

The new value-based healthcare environment requires every staff member to understand how his or her role affects the organization's success to enhance the patient experience, generate high-quality outcomes, and keep costs low. Human resource leaders, education professionals, and compliance officers design curricula for these classroom programs that offer hands-on exploration and deep understanding of topics related to the healthcare field in general and the business of healthcare specifically targeted at the regulatory environment that governs the hospital business. As a result, staff members can connect what they are learning to the rationale behind their specific job requirements, increasing their satisfaction with the training experience and adding to their ability to apply the information effectively.

Self-directed education

The rapidly changing landscape of federal and state rules and regulations requires a self-directed and motivated UR team to stay abreast of changing environmental expectations. It is wise to rely on department leaders to share relevant regulatory information, but it's even wiser to encourage staff members to independently seek resources that will keep their knowledge current. Point-of-entry utilization review and vigilant resource management allow hospitals to serve entire communities, including those who are uninsured or underinsured. These professionals also play an important role in containing healthcare costs, which preserves access to care for those who can't afford to pay for it out of pocket.

Many resources have been mentioned throughout this text, but some are of greater value than others. Here are some self-directed learning opportunities that we find to be of value. Many give the UR specialist the opportunity to access the latest information, ask questions, and receive clarification from peers and colleagues:

- American College of Physician Advisors offers a range of information for PAs and their colleagues. Worth budgeting for the modest $125 annual membership fee. *http://www.acpadvisors.org/*
- One of the most valuable resources for UR specialists is the Google Group RAC Relief. We urge readers to sign on to this free Q&A resource, which serves as an open forum for PAs and other revenue cycle specialists. *https://groups.google.com/u/1/g/rac-relief*
- *Finally Friday* is a biweekly open webinar that features seasoned panelists discussing timely topics of UR interest at 1–2 p.m. Eastern *https://www.myfinallyfriday.com/*
- Athena Forum Institute has been around for many years and has earned a position as provider of education for the Commission for Case Management Certification (CCMC) with a wide variety of hospital case management programs. *https://athenaforum.net*
- HCPro Medicare Boot Camp®—Utilization Review Version. Although Medicare focused, the information here is broad enough to apply to most commercial UR issues. *https://hcmarketplace.com/medicare-boot-camp-hospital-vrsn-1*
- *The Hospitalist* is the news magazine of the Society of Hospital Medicine and often has articles pertaining to the business of healthcare. *www.the-hospitalist.org*
- ICD10Monitor sponsors "Talk Ten Tuesdays," a half-hour weekly show featuring conversations on a variety of hospital business operations and current issues. *https://www.icd10monitor.com/talk-ten-tuesdays*

- RAC Monitor sponsors "Monitor Monday," a half-hour weekly show highlighting regulatory and audit news. *https://www.racmonitor.com/monitor-mondays/*

In addition, we maintain websites that readers may find of value. Dr. Hirsch's website is packed with detailed information on all things related to hospitals (*www.ronaldhirsch.com/*). Ms. Daniels' consulting company maintains a website featuring blog commentaries on hospital case management, utilization review, and related topics at *www.phoenixmed.net/*.

References

Allen, M. (2018). Unnecessary Medical Care Is More Common than You Think. ProPublica. Retrieved from *https://www.propublica.org/article/unnecessary-medical-care-is-more-common-than-you-think*.

American Case Management Association. (2019). 2019 National Hospital Case Management Survey Final Report. Retrieved from *https://www.acmaweb.org/2019_Survey/2019_NHCMS.pdf*.

Bagshaw, S. M., Tran D. T., Opgenorth, T., et al. (2020). Assessment of Costs of Avoidable Delays in Intensive Care Unit Discharge. *JAMA Network Open, 3*(8):e2013913.

Betbeze, P. (4 October 2013). Don't Expect Physicians to Lead Change. HealthLeaders. Retrieved from *http://www.healthleadersmedia.com/leadership/dont-expect-physicians-lead-change*.

Case Management Society of America. (2019). The Practice of Hospital Case Management: A White Paper. Little Rock, Arkansas.

Centers for Medicare & Medicaid Services. (CMS). (2011). Condition of Participation: Utilization Review. 42 *CFR 482.30*. Washington, DC. Retrieved from *https://www.gpo.gov/fdsys/granule/CFR-2011-title42-vol5/ CFR-2011-title42-vol5-sec482-30*.

CMS. (December 2020). NHE fact sheet. Retrieved from *https://www.cms.gov/Research-Statistics-Data-and-Systems/Statistics-Trends-and-Reports/NationalHealthExpendData/NHE-Fact-Sheet*.

Department of Justice. (14 January 2021). Justice Department Recovers Over $2.2 Billion from False Claims Act Cases in Fiscal Year 2020. Retrieved from *https://www.justice.gov/opa/pr/justice-department-recovers-over-22-billion-false-claims-act-cases-fiscal-year-2020*.

Department of Justice. (19 March 2021). 14 Defendants Sentenced to 74+ Years in Forest Park Healthcare Fraud. Retrieved from *https://www.justice.gov/usao-ndtx/pr/14-defendants-sentenced-74-years-forest-park-healthcare-fraud*.

Hsiao, W. C., Sapolsky, H. M., Dunn, D. L., & Weiner, S. L. (1986). Lessons of the New Jersey DRG Payment System. Health Affairs, 5(2). Retrieved from *https://www.healthaffairs.org/doi/abs/10.1377/hlthaff.5.2.32*.

Himmelstein, D. U., Thorne, D., Warren, E., and Woolhandler, S. (June 2009). Medical Bankruptcy in the United States, 2007: Results of a National Study. *The American Journal of Medicine, 122*(8), 741–746. Retrieved from *https://www.amjmed.com/article/S0002-93430900404-5/fulltext*.

IMS Institute for Healthcare Informatics. (2013). Avoidable Costs in U.S. Healthcare. Retrieved from *http://offers.premierinc.com/rs/381-NBB-525/images/Avoidable_Costs_in%20_US_Healthcare-IHII_ AvoidableCosts_2013%5B1%5D.pdf*.

Institute of Medicine. (2010). The Healthcare Imperative: Lowering Costs and Improving Outcomes. The National Academies Collection: Reports funded by National Institutes of Health. Washington, DC. Retrieved from *https://pubmed.ncbi.nlm.nih.gov/21595114/*.

KaufmanHall. (March 2021). National Hospital Flash Report. Retrived from *https://www.kaufmanhall.com/ ideas-resources/research-report/national-hospital-flash-report-summary-march-2021*.

Kacik, A. (2019). Health systems redefine training to re-energize employees. Modern Healthcare. Retrieved from *https://www.modernhealthcare.com/labor/health-systems-redefine-training-re-energize-employees*.

Krauss, G. (20 November 2017). Are best practices in CDI really best practices? ICD10 Monitor. Retrieved from *https://www.linkedin.com/pulse/best-practices-cdi-really-glenn-krauss/*.

Krauss, G. (26 August 2019). Maximizing or Optimizing: In search of a better approach to CDI. ICD10 Monitor. Retrieved from *https://www.icd10monitor.com/maximizing-or-optimizing-in-search-of-a-better-approach-to-cdi*.

Lyu, H. (2017). Overtreatment in the United States. PLoS One. Retrieved from *https://journals.plos.org/plosone/article?id=10.1371/journal.pone.0181970*.

McCarthy, A. (24 May 2017). Preventing unnecessary breast cancer treatment. Cancer Research UK Science Blog. Retrieved from *https://news.cancerresearchuk.org/2017/05/24/preventing-unnecessary-breast-cancer-treatment/*.

McDermott, K. W., Jiang H. J. (June 2020). Characteristics and Costs of Potentially Preventable Inpatient Stays, 2017. Agency for Healthcare Research and Quality, Rockville, MD. Retrieved from *www.hcup-us.ahrq.gov/reports/statbriefs/sb259-Potentially-Preventable-Hospitalizations-2017.pdf*.

Maguire, P. (May 2018). Physician advisors: Young Doctors Should Apply. Today's Hospitalist. Retrieved from *https://www.todayshospitalist.com/physician-advisors/*.

Martin, K. L. (2020). Medscape Hospitalist Compensation Report. Retrieved from *https://www.medscape.com/slideshow/2020-compensation-hospitalist-6013015*.

Page, L. (26 April 2016). Hospitalists: Riding the wave of changes in healthcare. Medscape. Retrieved from *https://www.medscape.com/viewarticle/861921*.

Ramey, M, & Daniels, S. (2005). *The Leader's Guide to Hospital Case Management*. Sudbury, MA: Jones & Bartlett Learning.

Saad, L. (2019). More Americans Delaying Medical Treatment Due to Cost. Gallup News. Retrieved from *https://news.gallup.com/poll/269138/americans-delaying-medical-treatment-due-cost.aspx*.

Shoemaker, W. (2019). Bad debt expense benchmarks: U.S. acute care hospitals show improvements since 2015. Retrieved from *https://www.hfma.org/topics/hfm/2019/october/bad-debt-expense-benchmarks-us-acute-care-hospitals-show-improvements.html*.

St. John, A. (2017). How the Affordable Care Act drove down personal bankruptcy. Consumer Reports. Retrieved from *https://www.consumerreports.org/personal-bankruptcy/how-the-aca-drove-down-personal-bankruptcy/*.

Sullivan, T. (18 June 2020). Integra's Health Care Fraud Lawsuit Against Baylor Scott & White Dismissed. Policy and Medicine. Retrieved from *https://www.policymed.com/2020/06/integras-health-care-fraud-lawsuit-against-baylor-scott-white-dismissed.html*.

Tahari, P. A., Butz, D. A., and Greenfield, L. J. (2000). Length of stay has minimal impact on the cost of hospital admission. *Journal of the American College of Surgeons, 191*(2):123–130.

CHAPTER 5

The Utilization Review Process: Pre-Admission and Admissions

The UR Process and a Front-End Revenue Cycle

The challenge of the future of healthcare comes down to three words: managing medical costs. As value-based payment plans spread across the country to medical practices and hospitals alike, the foundational elements of utilization review (UR), such as medical necessity, patient status, level of care, intensity of services, authorizations, denials, and outcomes, will all gain in importance as hospitals struggle to maintain healthy margins. Thus, it is prudent to have utilization review aligned and closely involved with the revenue cycle.

The Utilization Review Process

Different hospitals interpret UR in different ways. Some consider it a department; others may consider it a plan or an economic essential for a healthy revenue cycle. Whatever position your hospital takes, there is no doubt that UR has a direct impact on the financial health of the hospital, and tight collaboration between UR and the revenue cycle/finance department makes good sense.

Originally, UR was based on the physician's certification that the patient required a hospital level of care. But today, every insurer seeks detailed, individualized clinical information to justify the admission status, the level of care, and the prescribed treatment plan and a clear understanding that the services can be safely provided only at a hospital level of care. The content of the medical record is therefore critical to payers' understanding of why a patient needs hospitalization and whether the services prescribed are appropriate to the status and level of care. It's one thing to identify a clinical label (diagnosis) that describes the patient's status but quite another to capture the nuances of the patient's condition to convey a concise, complete, and accurate portrait of the patient's medical status at the initial point of entry, during treatment, and while preparing for recovery outside of the hospital. The UR process ensures the collection of information at these points in a patient's care to evaluate medical necessity and the appropriateness of care related to desired outcomes.

In this discussion about the nuances of these determinations, "status" will refer to the admission status of the patient, either inpatient or outpatient, whereas "level of care" will refer to the care setting within the hospital, such as a general medical unit, a step-down unit, or an intensive care unit. While many still refer to admission status as level of care, the changes implemented by The Centers for Medicare & Medicaid Services (CMS) in 2013 with the 2-midnight rule has blurred the lines between inpatient and outpatient as far as the intensity of care. For example, a patient can have an outpatient status and receive care in the intensive care unit.

The concept of "inpatient level of care" dates back prior to the adoption of the 2-midnight rule and was eliminated with its adoption. Interestingly, CMS' *Quality Improvement Organization (QIO) Manual,* Chapter 4, section 4110, as of the date of this book's publication, continues to state, "The patient must demonstrate signs and/or symptoms severe enough to warrant the need for medical care and must receive services of such intensity that they can be furnished safely and effectively only on an inpatient basis." It should be noted that this section, last updated 11 July 2003, is only applicable to reviews by the QIO, and, in our opinion, was an oversight by CMS and should be viewed as obsolete.

Understanding Medical Necessity

Because medical necessity plays a part in each stage of the UR process, we want to review essential information about medical necessary to help readers understand its applicability throughout the UR process. From clinical information to justify an outpatient service or inpatient admission to clinical information to defend a claim, medical necessity is often a deciding factor for claims payment. For better or worse, we have become accustomed to healthcare benefits being managed by insurers. As such, the language of medical necessity, which serves as the central concept within these systems, is very familiar. Some may say that the physician is in the best position to determine medical necessity. Although that's generally true, it must also be noted that health insurance is a defined benefit plan that covers only services specified in the policy. For example, no one would argue that seeing a dentist for a cavity is medically necessary, but dental care is generally not covered on medical policies. Other policies may have limitations such as not covering organ transplantation. And, as discussed elsewhere in this book, the medical standard of care is ever evolving, with new treatments for once untreatable diseases and new data showing that old treatments are no longer effective, which called a medical reversal. When a physician orders a medical service, it must be remembered that they are spending someone else's money on that service and the party that controls the money has a vested interest in ensuring the money is spent wisely.

Representatives of insurance companies are not present at the patient's bedside assessing their condition minute by minute and determining whether hospital care is warranted and which care is necessary and should be paid and which care is not necessary. The payer, and all others who will be caring for that patient, from nursing to nutritionists to pastoral services, count on the physicians, who are expected to convey a concise, complete, and accurate portrait of the patient's medical status at the initial point of entry, during treatment, and while preparing for recovery outside of the hospital. Until recently, with the escalation of prices, high-deductible plans, and underinsured patients, neither consumers nor their physicians were fully aware of the power of the term medical necessity to deny care. In fact, the idiosyncratic way that coverage decisions are made in healthcare organizations has led to variations that often create inequity for consumers, greater volume of denials and appeals, and more litigation.

The UR process is required to determine whether the care a physician provides to the patient is medically necessary, must be done in a hospital setting, is in the appropriate status, at what level of care, and is reimbursable by the payer. There is considerable variation in the way medical necessity is defined among insurers and government agencies, but §1862 (a)(1)(a) of the Social Security Act provides the basic groundwork, stating the following:

> *Notwithstanding any other provisions of this title, no payment may be made …for any expenses incurred for items or services, which are not reasonable and necessary for the diagnosis or treatment of illness or injury or to improve the functioning of a malformed body member.*

CMS and its Medicare contractors have long determined whether items and services are reasonable and necessary, either through the case-by-case review of the clinical appropriateness of claims or through local and national coverage policies, such as Local Coverage Determinations (LCD) and National Coverage Determinations (NCD). They have done so without this reasonable and necessary standard being specifically defined in regulations. But in January 2021, in association with a new rule on Medicare Coverage of Innovative Technology (MCIT), CMS finalized an expanded definition of reasonable and necessary Medicare coverage that will be used for coverage decisions (CMS-3372-F) but then delayed implementation of this rule with a new rule (CMS-3372-F2) to allow further comment and analysis (CMS, 18 May 2021).

The MCIT rule includes the following proposed factors for defining medical necessity:

- Factor 1: Safe and effective
- Factor 2: Not experimental or investigational (except for Category B Investigational Device Exemption devices)
- Factor 3: Appropriate for Medicare beneficiaries, including the duration and frequency that are considered appropriate for the item or service, in terms of whether it meets all of the following criteria:
  - Furnished in accordance with accepted standards of medical practice for the diagnosis or treatment of the patient's condition or to improve the function of a malformed body member
  - Furnished in a setting appropriate to the patient's medical needs and condition
  - Ordered and furnished by qualified personnel
  - Meets, but does not exceed, the patient's medical need
  - At least as beneficial as an existing and available medically appropriate alternative; *or*
  - Is covered by commercial insurers, unless evidence supports that differences between Medicare beneficiaries and commercially insured individuals are clinically relevant

Although most of these are similar to factors already found in Chapter 13 § 13.5.4 of CMS' *Payment Integrity Manual,* the final bullet point concerning commercial insurance coverage led to the delay. Many commenters noted that the commercial insurance patient population is distinct from the Medicare population and, therefore, a different standard may be appropriate. On 16 September, 2021, in CMS-3372-P2 the agency proposed to withdraw the MCIT proposed rule in its entirety based on concerns about commercial coverage and its applicability to Medicare beneficiaries. As of the time of this writing, the outcome is not known.

CMS does not consider the cost of care when making coverage decisions; it bases these decisions solely on nonfinancial considerations. Commercial insurers have generally adopted a similar definition but often add cost as a consideration. They compare the cost of the proposed service to that of other options that produce the same therapeutic or diagnostic results. For example, intensity-modulated radiation therapy (IMRT) can be used for treatment of radiosensitive cancers, providing added accuracy and potentially reduced risk of damage to nearby structures compared to traditional three-dimensional conformal radiation therapy—but at a higher cost. Therefore, when approving the use of the therapy, insurers will evaluate its relative effectiveness and safety, the benefits over three-dimensional conformal radiation therapy, and its cost. These decisions can get specific, as insurers may approve IMRT for treatment of breast cancer in the left breast, where radiation to the heart and surrounding structures can have adverse effects, but not for treatment of breast cancer in the right breast.

Documentation of medical necessity

Electronic health records (EHR) promised significant improvement in clinical documentation but brought new challenges to the industry. Notably, physicians and other clinicians have reported feeling burdened by the data entry demands of EHRs—responsibilities that take away from their time and focus on patients and are commonly cited as a source of physician burnout (Tajirian, 2020). It is not unusual to hear physicians refer to the EHR as a tool designed to improve billing accuracy but not improve patient care.

The dramatic increase in the quantity of information in the medical record has resulted in a marked decrease in the quality and utility of that information. Notes produced by EHRs are often many pages long and full of templated, check-the-box documentation. The overuse of copy and paste is one of the many workarounds clinicians employ to save time while documenting in the EHR. However, it creates voluminous and often imprecise notes, which muddles the story of the patient's course of care and makes it difficult for future readers, not to mention creating complications for coding and billing. Only 18% of text in inpatient progress notes are original entries by clinicians, according to a 2017 study conducted at UCSF Medical Center. The remaining 82% of text was copied or imported from another portion of the record (Wang, 2017).

Gaps in medical documentation have always been present, but once the link between medical documentation and hospital payment became a critical factor in ensuring a continuous revenue stream, hospital leaders took some innovative steps to make sure that all the t's are crossed and the i's are dotted. At some larger facilities, for example, financial officers have set up division-specific revenue cycle processes, and all cases are reviewed post-authorization within each division, ensuring that all the necessary pieces of information are in the record before a patient is actually hospitalized.

CMS has stated that the physician's "order and certification regarding medical necessity" are not entitled to any "presumptive weight" and are "evaluated in the context of the evidence in the medical record" (42 *CFR* §412.46[b]). Unfortunately, cloned records rarely contain useful information to assist QIO, Recovery Audit Contractors, or commercial auditors in ascertaining the reason for hospitalization or inpatient admission, or—more importantly—to assist other caregivers in understanding the physician's thinking, concerns, and plans for the patient.

Physicians should be encouraged to "think in ink." The use of check boxes and templates does work well in some cases, such as for documentation of the past medical history, review of systems, and physical examination. However, the history of present illness (HPI) and the assessment and treatment plan are unique to each patient, and a template should not be used when documenting this information in the record. These sections of the chart paint the picture of a patient's medical condition and allow a clinician or reviewer to better understand the need for hospital care. This same "portrait" may be reviewed months or years down the line, and a lack of narrative order often impedes clarity. Complete documentation also allows the hospital to accurately capture the patient's comorbidities, complications, and conditions present on admission, which helps the coding process and promotes accurate risk adjustments. By writing a narrative instead of using a template or check boxes, the physician has the opportunity to elaborate on his or her medical decision-making (MDM), a crucial component of physician coding and billing.

Experts advise that documentation of medical necessity to justify acute care should demonstrate the complexities of MDM and should begin with the patient's chief complaint, acuity of the patient's condition, any comorbidities, why the nature of the patient's condition warrants hospital level of care, and the potential risks if the patient is not admitted. These four points—and their mnemonic HOPE—may be helpful to the physician-coaching process.

1. **History and physical** or **HPI** if in the emergency department (ED) and patient throughput is a priority
2. **Orders** for a treatment plan with services and procedures that can only be safely provided at a hospital level of care
3. **Potential** risk if patient is not treated in the hospital
4. **Expectation** of at least a 2-midnight stay in the hospital via a "Because" clause

CMS stated in the 2014 Inpatient Prospective Payment System (IPPS) final rule that it expects providers to clearly document the need for hospitalization, including the risks and their plans for the patient:

The factors that lead a physician to admit a particular beneficiary based on the physician's clinical expectation are significant clinical considerations and must be clearly and completely documented in the medical record. Because of the relationship that develops between a physician and his or her patient, the physician is in a unique position to incorporate complete medical evidence in a beneficiary's medical records, and has ample opportunity to explain in detail why the expectation of the need for care spanning at least two midnights was appropriate in the context of that beneficiary's acute condition. (CMS, 2013)

In 2021, new guidelines for selection of evaluation and management codes in the office setting were adopted that allow code selection based on total time spent or MDM. It is hoped that this will limit the amount of superfluous documentation that is added to meet the coding guidelines. It is believed that these guidelines will expand to be applicable to the hospital setting in the near future.

Admission order as condition of payment

When first written and adopted in 2013, the 2-midnight rule added to the regulations a condition of payment that required an inpatient admission order provided by a physician with admitting privileges and *authenticated prior to discharge*. Many providers saw an immediate uptick in technical denials with no opportunity to appeal and no review to determine if the admission otherwise was appropriate for Part A payment. Once CMS realized what was happening, they removed a signed admission order before discharge as a condition of payment, a change that became effective October 1, 2018. When the revision was initially proposed, CMS clearly stated that it never intended that the "admission order documentation requirements should by themselves lead to the denial of payment for otherwise medically reasonable and necessary inpatient stays" (Hirsch, 2018).

With this 2018 clarification removing an authenticated admission order as a condition of payment, revenue cycle personnel should submit claims whether or not the admission order was signed at the time of claim submission. But as with many changes in regulation, dissemination to the key hospital personnel was variable. Some organizations assumed that an admission order was not needed at all and put themselves in denial jeopardy, while at other organizations billers continued to self-deny if the admission order was absent or not authenticated at the time of discharge. As of this writing, most organization have adopted compliant processes that support efficient claims submission and follow-up of missing or incomplete admission order, but it remains a cautionary tale about how rules are interpreted.

It should also be noted that CMS clarified in Chapter 1 of the *Medicare Benefit Policy Manual* that in extremely rare circumstances, an inpatient admission can be billed to Part A in the absence of an admission order if the intent of the physician to admit the patient is clear and there was no reasonable possibility that the care could have been adequately provided in an outpatient setting.

The Four Stages of the UR Process

The UR process can be organized in four stages: pre-admission, admission, concurrent, and post-acute. The process may also be described as occurring before, during, or after care is provided. The decision of when to initiate the UR process is driven partly by the payer, partly by logistics, and partly by the political will of the executive team. The C-suite must support efforts to get it right the first time to avoid rework, back-end fixes, and loss of revenue due to payer denials. Most commercial insurers require precertification of elective care and prompt notification of emergent hospital care, whereas Medicare allows the UR process to be prospective, concurrent, and retrospective depending on the hospital's UR policy, as required by the *Conditions of Participation* (*CoP*), and depending on the availability of staff to perform the review and act on the result. This section will focus on the first two stages of the UR process: prospective/pre-admission review—generally reserved for elective, transfer, and direct admissions—and admission review, which is reserved for emergency department admissions. Together, these activities are often referred to as access management. A robust access management program will demonstrate the financial value of a front-end revenue cycle model that operates at lower cost than traditional back-end revenue cycle models. That's why we take the position that the prospective UR process as part of a front-end revenue cycle is the most effective operational model.

Stage 1: Prospective/pre-admission review

Prospective review refers to the activities designed to confirm that the care planned for the patient is both medically necessary and covered by the payer *prior to the care being provided.*

There are typically two components of the prospective review process. The first includes all activities required to identify the patient, capture the billing information necessary for claims processing, and confirm benefit eligibility. This allows for adequate time to obtain the necessary information, contact the payer, or review the information in relation to published coverage guidelines. Basic information, including the patient's demographics, insurance information, and diagnoses, is always required for precertification. Commercial insurers often use third-party companies to perform UR. Depending on the care that is precertified, these companies may require extensive clinical information, such as prior care provided to the patient, results of previous laboratory testing and imaging, current medications, and pertinent physical examination findings. For this reason, it is best for the ordering physician and the physician's staff to complete the pre-certification for procedures. It is also crucial that this documentation gets incorporated into the hospital medical record. While the office records may support justification for a procedure, if the hospital claim is audited and those clinical records are not part of the medical record sent to the payer, a denial is likely. The physician need not prepare new documentation to meet this requirement; the office notes can simply be incorporated into the hospital medical record as an electronic attachment.

The second component includes the activities to confirm medical necessity. The determination of medical necessity is discussed elsewhere in this book.

Administrative activities

The first step of the prospective review process is generally delegated to clerical/support personnel in access management or the admissions office who can forward demographic and preliminary diagnostic information to the payer, whereas the second step benefits from a trained UR specialist, often known as the access review specialist (ARS), who has the clinical expertise to provide more detailed information and answer payer queries about indications, past testing, test results, and so on. For elective tests, procedures, and requests for a hospital bed—inpatient or outpatient/observation—the process should begin as soon as the care is scheduled or the need for care is confirmed. As part of this process, payers may also request some clinical information reflecting the patient's current medical status, and they may preauthorize the care.

Administrative activities include the essential revenue cycle activities to ensure that the demographic information concerning patients' identity, health insurance confirmation, coverage benefits, and personal information is current and correct. Based on personal experience, we can report that UR and/or care coordinators report that demographic, or face sheet, information is incomplete or inaccurate upwards of 40% of the time. These professionals often must stop what they're doing to correct demographic information, but this does not solve the problem at the source.

As a reminder to the administrative team, there are only two recognized statuses: inpatient and outpatient. It is not uncommon to hear reference to patients who are being placed in observation, as if observation were a status. It is not. Observation is a service provided to outpatients with a physician order for observation. In practical terms, if a doctor orders "observation" as the patient's admission status, that can be regarded as an order for outpatient status with observation services.

Precertification for elective services

As more physician practices are acquired by hospitals and health systems, precertification is often centralized, with the hospital UR staff remotely accessing the physician's electronic medical record or, in some areas, obtaining the needed information via fax. The precertification information, along with the clinical information that led to the approval, is incorporated into the hospital medical record, as this information is clinically useful when caring for the patient during hospitalization and is often required if the medical record is audited retrospectively. See Figure 5.1 for an example of precertification.

■ Figure 5.1

Precertification case example

The MitraClip is an FDA-approved medical device that is used to treat severe mitral regurgitation in patients who are deemed to be at prohibitive risk for surgery. The MitraClip is placed percutaneously via a catheter threaded into the heart from the femoral vein.

The MitraClip is covered for Medicare patients (both traditional and MA) if the requirements of the coverage decision memo, issued August 7, 2014, are met. However, coverage varies if the patient is insured by a commercial insurer. For patients insured by United HealthCare, MitraClip is noncovered per their coverage policy. According to the policy, "There is insufficient evidence in the clinical literature demonstrating the long-term efficacy of catheter-delivered mitral valve prostheses for treating mitral disease." For patients insured by Aetna, MitraClip is considered medically necessary "for persons with grade 3+ to 4+ symptomatic degenerative mitral regurgitation and at high-risk for traditional open-heart mitral valve surgery."

UR staff who review cardiac procedures and physicians who perform the MitraClip procedure must be aware that it is crucial to determine the correct insurance coverage and requirements for MitraClip before discussing the procedure with the patient. Note that lack of coverage does not mean that the procedure cannot be performed—it only means that the payer will not pay for it.

Source: Transcatheter heart valve procedures, Policy Number: 2018T0557N, from www.uhcprovider.com/content/dam/provider/docs/public/policies/comm-medical-drug/transcatheter-heart-valve-procedures.pdf; percutaneous mitral valve repair from www.aetna.com/cpb/medical/data/800_899/0880.html.

Commercial payers generally demand more clinical information if precertification is for a procedure or surgery that will require a stay in the hospital. If the payer is a Medicare Advantage (MA) insurer, it will want even more clinical information than its commercial counterparts, as MA insurers receive a risk-adjusted payment (see Chapter 2 for more detailed information on risk adjustment) and thus will want all information that can be compliantly coded as comorbidities and may affect the patient's risk adjustment score. This may explain why commercial payers often prefer telephonic reviews for their MA members, which offer the opportunity to ask more questions about the clinical status of the patient than what would normally be included in a transmitted InterQual® or MCG Care Guidelines report.

Clinical activities

Physicians must document medical necessity, which must be confirmed by the ARS, regardless of whether the hospital works with MA or other commercial payers. Typically, the insurance company will indicate how many days of hospitalization are approved and at what point, if any, the insurer requires continued-stay authorization. Some insurance plans also specify the number of days that are approved at each level of care—including intensive care, monitored, and general medical-surgical—and adherence to this approval is crucial if the hospital is paid per diem at variable rates depending on the level of care. The precertification contact, whether done by phone or electronically, should also obtain the following:

- Authorization for any potential post-hospital services that may be required (e.g., approval for a stay in a skilled nursing facility [SNF] or home care services after joint replacement surgery)
- A list of approved providers to streamline the transition process after the patient is hospitalized
- The names of any payer contacts that may be needed by the case manager or UR specialist during the course of the patient's hospitalization

Many insurance companies provide their coverage guidelines online in a provider manual. Updates are performed frequently as the medical literature and evidence of effectiveness change and as new procedures, tests, and medications are developed and approved for use. Likewise, CMS has developed the Medicare Coverage Database (*www.cms.gov/mcd*), where providers can find current, proposed, and future NCDs and LCDs. Providers should use these websites as primary sources, because a printed copy of a manual may include an out-of-date policy and complying with it may result in denial of payment of the claim. In 2021, CMS refreshed the Medicare Coverage Database website, making it significantly easier to use and find applicable documents.

Medicare inpatient-only list

CMS publishes a yearly inpatient-only list, also known as Addendum E, citing surgeries that surgeons must perform on an inpatient basis if they are to be reimbursed by Medicare. Each year, as part of the Outpatient Prospective Payment System (OPPS) rulemaking process, CMS reviews all new procedures for inclusion on the inpatient-only list and reviews all surgeries currently on the list for removal. To determine whether procedures should be removed from the list, CMS reviews them based on the following four criteria:

1. Most outpatient departments are equipped to provide the services to the Medicare population

2. The simplest procedure described by the code may be performed in most outpatient departments

3. The procedure is related to codes that have already been removed from the inpatient list

4. The procedure is being performed in numerous hospitals on an outpatient basis

CMS has made it clear that removal of a surgery from the inpatient-only list does not mean that it must be performed as outpatient. CMS expects physicians to use their clinical judgment and the guidelines established in the 2-midnight rule to determine the proper admission status for all patients whose planned surgery is not on the inpatient-only list.

In the 2021 OPPS final rule, CMS announced that beginning January 1, 2021, and over the next three years, it would gradually eliminate the inpatient-only list. Starting with about 300 musculoskeletal-related services in 2021, CMS stated that the elimination of the list would make the services payable when furnished in the hospital outpatient setting when outpatient care is appropriate. As this book was in the editing process, CMS released the 2022 OPPS proposed rule, which included a proposal to reverse the policy eliminating the inpatient-only list and placing the 298 surgeries removed from the list in 2021 back on the list for 2022. According to the 2022 OPPS proposed rule, a more gradual approach will be used to remove surgeries in the future (CMS, 19 July 2021). The 2022 OPPS final rule and decision about the reversal will not be published prior to publication of this book. Readers should understand that the concepts discussed in this section will continue to apply to surgeries that are removed from the inpatient-only list, either individually or in groups.

CMS also stated in 2020 that it intends to add more services to the list of procedures approved to be performed at ambulatory surgical centers (ASC) under new criteria finalized in the 2021 ASC final rule (CMS, 2020). CMS is required by law to publish the inpatient-only surgery list and the ASC-approved surgery list at least 60 days prior to January 1 of each year as Addendum E and Addendum AA, respectively, to the OPPS final rule.

Procedures are listed on the addenda by their Healthcare Common Procedure Coding System (HCPCS) code and short descriptor. These codes are also known as the Level II Current Procedural Terminology (CPT®) codes, which are copyrighted by the American Medical Association and cannot be used without permission. Because of the coding, hospital coders use ICD-10-PCS when billing for inpatient surgeries, whereas physicians use HCPCS/CPT codes when scheduling and billing surgery. Unfortunately, there is no direct crosswalk between the HCPCS codes and the corresponding ICD-10-PCS codes. As a result, a physician may correctly schedule a procedure as inpatient based on a HCPCS code that is on the inpatient-only list. Subsequently, the hospital coding staff will code the procedure by using the most appropriate ICD-10-PCS code and billing with that code. But when reviewed by the Medicare Administrative Contractor, the ICD-10-PCS codes are converted back to HCPCS codes. In many cases, the new HCPCS code is not the same one that was used to schedule the surgery, and if this new code does not have the same status as the original code, a denial for incorrect admission status can result.

Commercial insurers (including MA plans) may choose to follow the codes on the CMS inpatient-only list, use the inpatient lists provided in commercial level of care guidelines (i.e., InterQual or MCG Care Guidelines), or develop their own proprietary list. This bizarre coding arrangement may explain why many denials are overturned once the coding staff explain the discrepancies via an appeal letter. This also creates confusion for physicians who may be asked to order a different admission status for similar patients undergoing the same surgery.

Inpatient or outpatient surgery?

When a procedure is removed from the inpatient-only list, there may be confusion about how to apply admission status determinations. For example, CMS removed total knee arthroplasty (TKA) from the inpatient-only list in 2018. In the 2018 OPPS final rule commentary, CMS indicated that the admission status of such patients should follow the 2-midnight rule, including the use of the "case-by-case" exception. Because TKA is an elective procedure, these patients do not have life-threatening illnesses and thus do not fit the examples provided by the BFCC-QIOs when the case-by-case exception to the 2-midnight rule was introduced in 2016. However, many of these patients do have several comorbid conditions that increase both their perioperative risk and the chance of an adverse event happening to the patient during their surgery and hospital stay. Thus, in the 2018 OPPS final rule commentary, CMS made several statements suggesting that patients at higher surgical risk could be admitted as inpatient regardless of the expected LOS. CMS stated the following:

> We believe that there is a subset of less medically complex TKA cases that could be appropriately and safely performed on an outpatient basis. However, we do not expect a significant volume of TKA cases currently being performed in the hospital inpatient setting to shift to the hospital outpatient setting as a result of removing this procedure from the inpatient-only list. At this time, we expect that a significant number of Medicare beneficiaries will continue to receive treatment as an inpatient for TKA procedures. (CMS, 14 December 2017)

The determination of risk is a subjective determination made by the physician. And as with other decisions, the determination must be supported by documentation in the medical record. Despite being asked, CMS has not released guidelines for determining which patients are at higher risk and warrant inpatient admission. It is therefore advised that every facility review the available guidance and develop guidelines for use by their medical staff using a multidisciplinary approach with input from surgeons, hospitalists, anesthesiologists, utilization management, compliance, and finance. Since the admission decision will be based on the perioperative risk to the patient, the admission order should be obtained prior to the start of surgery.

A subset of patients who undergo TKA will require care at a SNF after discharge from the hospital, either because of their physical condition and need for more intensive therapy than can be provided at home or because of the lack of caregivers at home. CMS noted in the final rule that this need could also be considered in the admission decision, stating that "the physician should take the beneficiaries' need for post-surgical services into account when selecting the site of care to perform the surgery."

In 2020, CMS removed total hip arthroplasty from the inpatient-only list. The same status determination paradigm applied to this surgery and again in 2021 when CMS removed 298 surgeries, predominantly orthopedic and spine surgeries, from the inpatient-only list. The end of 2020 and the first half of 2021 was a time of great confusion in hospitals around the country as they formulated policies and procedures for getting compliant status determinations on these surgeries and planning for the eventual abolition of the inpatient-only list in total. The announcement by CMS, noted above, that they are reversing course resulted in a great sigh of relief but also confusion about how to determine status for surgeries for the remainder of 2021.

Billing for inpatient-only cases

Hospitals cannot bill Medicare for an inpatient-only surgery on an outpatient claim and cannot change the admission status of a fee-for-service Medicare patient retroactively (except for condition code 44 changes) while the patient is hospitalized or after discharge. However, commercial insurers—and recall that MA is a commercial insurer and must be treated accordingly—may allow a hospital to retroactively change the billing status to meet their requirements; this change does not require a physician's order. In fact, UR specialists should avoid requesting an order from a physician under such circumstances, as doing so may lead the physician to generalize misleading information to Medicare patients and result in the physician unilaterally making status changes without consulting the UR staff. Also note that a higher level of care does not always result in a higher reimbursement, so UR staff should be wary of insurers that ask the hospital billing department representative to upgrade a patient from outpatient to inpatient after discharge. In this instance, UR staff should consult their finance counterparts and the payer's contract before authorizing such a change.

Medicare patients are not considered to be inpatient unless they are formally admitted as inpatients, with a valid order provided by a physician or other practitioner who is authorized by hospital rules and regulations and state law to admit patients to the hospital. Therefore, the admission order prior to a scheduled inpatient-only surgery should be obtained preoperatively.

However, on 1 April 2015, in a significant reversal of this long-standing policy, CMS issued guidance widening the use of the three-day payment window (CMS, 2015b). This allowed hospitals to bill for inpatient-only surgeries if the admission order is written at any time on the day of surgery or within the next three calendar days, as long as the patient is still hospitalized. It should be noted that although the inpatient order written in the three days after the surgery will allow the surgery to be billed on the inpatient claim and paid, the inpatient admission does not begin until the day the admission order is given. If the patient requires care in a skilled nursing facility, the counting for eligibility begins on the day of the admission order and not on the day of surgery.

Given the persistent confusion regarding inpatient-only list regulations (and based on best-practice observations by the authors), inpatient-only procedure confirmation should be resolved at the time of scheduling. Delaying the confirmation adds avoidable steps to the registration process and could place the hospital at financial risk. This preoperative review also allows the review of complete documentation of medical necessity for the planned procedure and allows the three-day clock for qualification for Part A SNF benefits to begin on the day of the inpatient-only surgery. Review in the recovery room will allow capture of the admission order on the first day but will result in some surgeries being performed without proper medical necessity documentation, thus risking a denial. Note that the standard in-hospital recovery for many surgeries exceeds the three-day window, so if the hospital adopts a policy of screening for proper admission status postoperatively, the screening should be performed as soon as possible and should not be delayed until discharge.

Elective medical admissions

Hospitals should also evaluate elective medical admissions for precertification prior to admission. Medicare does not have such a process to authorize the admission. However, if a procedure is planned during the admission, the hospital should review the appropriate NCD, LCD, or medical society guidelines to ensure medical necessity is met. If the admission is for administration of chemotherapy or other infusions such as intravenous antibiotics or pheresis, guidelines such as the National Comprehensive Cancer Network, Infectious Disease Society of America, or American Society for Apheresis should be consulted to ensure that the treatment meets the standard of care and requirements for medical necessity. This review should include obtaining office records from the physician and incorporating them into the hospital medical record to ensure that they are available for audit if necessary. As with surgeries, getting an approved length of stay (LOS) from the insurer and ensuring that the correct admission status was authorized confirms that the UR staff is alert to the need to provide the insurer with continued-stay reviews once the patient is hospitalized.

Transfer patients

Requests for transfer to access services that cannot be provided at an originating facility remain popular in today's marketplace of frequent mergers and acquisitions. Eliminating high-cost/low-revenue services in smaller hospitals means more frequent transfers to flagship hospitals in consolidated systems. Our nation's critical access hospitals also provide crucial medical services in rural communities whose size could not support a large medical center. These hospitals may be required to transfer patients with complex illnesses or injuries to regional medical centers with the necessary expertise.

Best practice requires direct communication between the transferring and receiving facilities to share complete information on the patient's clinical condition, treatment given, reasons for transfer, mode of transfer, and timeline of requested transfer. This process is often undertaken by a dedicated team in access management to streamline the process and make it attractive to outlying hospitals. The ARS dedicated to manage the transfers is the lead point person to communicate with the originating facility to confirm that the receiving facility can provide the procedure or subspecialty requested. The ARS will also contact the on-call physician, requested specialist, or admitting hospitalist so that the physicians can consult personally before agreeing to the transfer. Subsequently, the ARS will arrange to receive necessary documents from the transferring facility and inform the relevant personnel of the case and anticipated treatment plan.

UR veterans know that patients transferred into their hospitals from facilities both near and far often have transition challenges, which become problems that the receiving hospital will have to resolve. As a result, formal transfer agreements have become routine. Except in the case of an emergency transfer, these agreements state that the originating facility agrees to accept the patient back once the specialty services of the accepting facility have been provided and completed and the patient is stable for transfer. These agreements also benefit the patient in that the originating hospital is best positioned to make post-acute care arrangements with a better understanding of the resources and providers available in the patient's hometown. An example of a transfer agreement appears in Figure 5.2.

■ **Figure 5.2**

Sample transfer agreement

Transfer agreement

From: (Receiving hospital) Community Hospital and Dr._____

To: (Transferring hospital) Community Hospital and Dr._____

Re: Patient: _____

Community Hospital agrees to admit the above-named patient being referred from _____ Medical Center/Hospital to receive specialized services of Dr. _____ for:

        _____ Diagnostic evaluation and consultation

        _____ Surgery

        _____ Treatment

        _____ Other

Specify: _____

Please note: When the patient has been deemed by the accepting Community Hospital and the receiving physician to be medically stable and/or treatable and no longer requires the highly specialized services of Community Hospital, the patient will be returned to the sending facility if discharge is not possible. This agreement includes the return for resolution of discharge barriers as well as continued acute care of a less specialized nature.

Direct referral for hospital care

The trend in using direct admissions seems to be abating, although it's still offered as a convenience to community primary care physicians (PCP) and is often viewed as a marketing opportunity for tertiary centers. However, the practice of accepting direct admissions presents some risk, and many hospitals have banned direct admissions altogether for reasons such as the following:

- A medical issue that turns out to be a social issue
- Patient shows up sicker than represented
- Unfamiliarity with PCP
- Uncertain diagnosis and unstable condition

Direct admissions should use the same process as elective admissions. Documentation from the PCP confirming medical necessity must be reviewed before the patient is referred to the hospital. Basic demographic and insurance information must be obtained, and there must be confirmation of acceptance by the on-call or admitting hospitalist or by the PCP if he or she will be the individual responsible for the patient's care. If the hospital is out of network with the patient's insurance, the patient and PCP should be notified to determine if it would be appropriate to contact the insurer and make arrangements for hospitalization at an in-network facility or obtain authorization from the insurer. With the ever-increasing use of hospitalists and absence of in-hospital PCPs who are up to date on hospital utilization regulations, a referral of a patient from a PCP for direct admission should no longer be considered evidence of the need for inpatient admission. The PCP is actually making a "direct referral for hospital care," and the admission status of the patient should not be determined until the patient arrives at the hospital and is evaluated. If it is determined that the patient is appropriate for outpatient status with observation services, the HCPCS code G0379 should be placed on the claim to indicate to CMS that the patient was referred directly from a community physician and not seen in the emergency department. For Medicare claims, the lack of G0379 or an emergency department visit code on the claim will result in nonpayment for the observation services.

Stage 2: Access management and emergency department admissions

Timely, concurrent review by the ARS staff is essential when a physician is considering hospitalizing a patient from the ED. In view of the increasing denials for inappropriate hospital admission status, the growing risk of fraud and abuse cases due to a lack of documentation for an inpatient admission, and recognition by hospital leaders of the costs associated with back-end fixes, rework, and the appeal process, hospital executives and UR directors are taking steps to begin the medical necessity determination process at the point of entry. How the process is structured depends upon the organization's size and available resources. In smaller facilities, an ARS or clinical documentation integrity team member may be colocated between the admissions office and the ED, while in larger facilities there may be a dedicated reviewer in both areas. However structured, there is no stopping the front-end revenue cycle trend as hospital leaders take steps to preserve revenue.

The recent announcement that some insurers will attempt to not pay for nonemergent ED visits has also prompted some innovative practices. In some hospitals, patients undergo an Emergency Medical Treatment and Active Labor Act medical screening before they cross the threshold into the ED clinical area. Those identified as nonemergent may be immediately referred to a clinic run by the hospital, an affiliated urgent care center, a medical home, or even a hospital-owned or affiliated primary physician's office or clinic where a block of time is carved out for walk-in appointments. The ability of insurers to deny such claims is now called into question by recent legislation, although it is expected that the insurers will continue to carefully scrutinize such claims.

There are often several different entry points through which a patient can get into a hospital bed. Referrals for admission can come from the ED, outpatient infusion center, cardiac catheterization lab, outpatient dialysis unit, hospital operating room, ambulatory surgery center, etc. For that reason, there has to be a consistent process to manage these requests no matter what the diagnosis or who the referring physician. Concurrent review allows the reviewer to collaborate in real time with the ED physician, referring physician, and/or admitting hospitalist to confirm that the care is medically necessary and provided at the proper level and the correct status is ordered. The ARS should be scanning the ED environment, checking the census board, and speaking with the nurses to identify potential admissions even before the physician determines the need for hospital care. The ARS will therefore be cognizant of the patient's status and can use the HOPE documentation mnemonic to remind the admitting physician to capture the salient points of the patient's immediate needs and the reason for an admission or placement as outpatient with observation.

The availability of an ARS in the ED also helps alleviate one of the most common and frustrating occurrences of a physician telling a patient they are being admitted to the hospital and then the patient is actually placed as outpatient. With an ARS present in the ED, the physicians can be told to discuss the need for hospital care with the patient but make no comment on status until they have discussed the case details with the ARS and the admitting physician to determine the correct admission status. This is also an opportunity to determine whether the patient is out of network, and, if so, transfer to an in-network facility should be considered if the patient is stable enough for such a move.

Concurrent review also provides an opportunity to speak with the patient and/or family to collect some background information that may help identify alternative options for the family and physician to consider. For example, if the patient was discharged within the past 30 days, a direct admission to a SNF might be clinically appropriate. The patient might only need a same-day home health visit, which could be immediately arranged. There are also several issues that the ARS must consider and share with the admitting medical team, such as a reminder about the parameters of the 2-midnight rule. Any issues that could affect the patient's discharge needs, including the social determinants of health, can be ascertained and passed on to the staff who will be involved in planning post-acute care.

Using screening tools

Hospital UR staff generally use screening tools, such as InterQual and MCG Care Guidelines, to help determine the need for hospitalization, the appropriate level of care placement within the hospital, and the correct admission status. Many insurers use these same tools for their reviews, although some will use modified proprietary versions. As part of the contract negotiations, make sure that the contract cites which tool is going to be used, and ensure that it includes a statement that if the insurer decides to change tools during the term of the contract, they must notify the point person cited on the contract in writing at least two weeks in advance of the change and permit the changes to be reviewed and negotiated.

Although they are not managed or required for use by CMS regulations, such tools have great value for the hospital reviewers. To use them with the 2-midnight rule, one must realize that the *first step is solely to determine whether hospital care itself is required*. If patients pass screening criteria, that means they most likely require hospital care, but the medical documentation must confirm this determination. This is a key distinction that was lost in the confusion surrounding the introduction of the 2-midnight rule. The next step is to determine how long the patient is expected to need hospital care, but this question cannot be answered by the screening tools as they are currently written. For example, the screening criteria would most likely determine that a patient who presents after a transient ischemic attack (TIA) and has many high-risk indicators will require an inpatient level of care. But if the physician's plan is to hospitalize the patient for 24 hours of neurologic monitoring and testing, then the patient does not warrant inpatient admission. Conversely, a patient who does not pass screening criteria may still require hospitalization. It's all in the documentation!

InterQual and MCG Care Guidelines both specify that their screening criteria are not all-encompassing, and cases that fail criteria screening should be sent for secondary review by a physician (the PA or member of the UR committee) if the ARS conversation with the admitting physician does not result in documentation improvement. In addition, a CMS notice from 2014, "Reviewing Hospital Claims for Patient Status," provides additional notes on medical necessity screening criteria as follows:

> It is not necessary for a beneficiary to meet an inpatient "level of care," as may be defined by a commercial screening tool, in order for Part A payment to be appropriate. In addition, meeting an inpatient "level of care," as may be defined by a commercial screening tool, does not make Part A payment appropriate in the absence of an expected LOS of two or more midnights. (CMS, March 2014)

Screening criteria is highly reliable and identifies the likelihood that hospital care is necessary. But experience has proven that the final determination of whether the hospital gets paid rests squarely with the physician's documentation. Let's be very clear about this: CMS does not require that you use specific screening criteria. In all cases, in addition to screening instruments, the reviewer applies his or her own clinical judgment to make a medical review determination based on the documentation in the medical record. The question of criteria use for Medicare contractors (or MA plans) and other commercial payers is fully dependent on the terms of the contract or provider manual. If they are silent on these issues, then the hospital has little recourse except to abide by the payer's demands.

Concurrent review and the PA

The roles and responsibilities of physician advisors (PA) were reviewed in Chapter 4, but the PA's involvement in the review process warrants additional commentary. As noted previously, determining the correct admission status for a patient is a two-step process. A first-level review by the UR specialist is standard. A second review by a PA occurs if admission documentation does not support inpatient status and the admitting physician is unable or unwilling to provide supporting information at the request of the UR specialist. In all cases, the UR specialist is expected to enter into a conversation with the admitting/attending physician to try to resolve the inconsistency before referring the case to the PA.

The PA may also get involved if documentation supports the guidelines but the status ordered (inpatient or outpatient) does not match the anticipated LOS and treatment plans for the patient. Screening criteria by itself, despite its comprehensive nature, cannot account for all patient scenarios, and the physician's documentation must be given consideration.

In the case of documentation that does not support screening criteria, the PA performing secondary review must evaluate the information in the medical record and determine whether hospitalization is clinically indicated. There are many available risk calculators that PAs can use to help make these decisions, such as the history, electrocardiogram, age, risk factors, and initial troponin scoring system for patients with chest pain; the Pneumonia Severity Index or CURB-65 criteria for community-acquired pneumonia; and the ABCD2 score for patients with TIA. These scoring tools are not all-inclusive, and medical research often leads to adjustment in the criteria; hence, the PA must use these tools along with the other nonquantifiable factors to determine whether hospitalization is medically necessary.

If hospital care is indicated, the PA should document his or her rationale in the UR system for future reference in case the hospital stay is later denied. If the PA determines that the physician's documentation does not indicate the need for hospitalization, then the PA should speak with the physician to determine whether there are undocumented factors that contributed to the physician's decision to hospitalize the patient. Any gaps in documentation must be amended accordingly. If agreement is not reached, then it may be appropriate to issue an Advance Beneficiary Notice or Hospital-Issued Notice of Non-Coverage as applicable for Medicare patients.

It is no longer mandated to assess the risk of an adverse event before deciding to hospitalize the patient. However, it may be useful only if that risk assessment applies to the time frame in question. For example, the ABCD2 score assesses the 48-hour risk of a stroke. Although a patient with a high score requires hospitalization, an inpatient admission would only be appropriate if the physician's plan is to keep the patient hospitalized for 48 hours after presentation. Likewise, in a patient with chest pain, the Thrombolysis in Myocardial Infarction score calculates the 14-day risk of an acute cardiac event, so a high score is helpful for deciding to hospitalize the patient for evaluation. However, the physician should be able to perform that evaluation in less than two midnights, so inpatient admission is not indicated.

When reviewing such cases, the PA should consider the normal course of the disease process, evidence-based treatment recommendations, and the patient's prior hospitalizations and response to treatment. In many cases, the decision is simple: A patient with septic shock or acute respiratory failure will require more than two midnights of care, and a patient with chest pain or syncope should require less than two midnights of care.

However, a substantial number of patients will fall into the area in between, which is why it is crucial to document the severity of the patient's presentation. A patient with an acute exacerbation of systolic heart failure who is also tachycardic and hypotensive is going to require a longer hospitalization than a patient who has heart failure and normal vital signs. Although vital signs are recorded elsewhere in the medical record, including them in the physician notes indicates that they were taken into account when selecting the correct admission status. In addition, such documentation allows the abnormal results to be coded as a comorbidity and establishes that it was present on admission—two important coding considerations.

The PA should provide feedback to the physician on the quality of his or her documentation and the accuracy of admission decisions while looking for evidence of overuse of inpatient admission or outpatient with observation services. By working together, the PA and physicians can ensure that every patient gets placed in the correct status every time.

Evidence-based protocols

If InterQual and MCG Care Guidelines represent evidence collected from the medical literature, then best-practice protocols represent the source documents. The use of scientifically sound algorithms, clinical practice guidelines, or practice protocols, such as those maintained by the Agency for Healthcare Research and Quality, is becoming more common as the pressure increases to reduce wasteful or excessive costs in preparation for value-based payments.

Several long-standing issues and new developments have contributed to this growing attention. First, decades of outcome studies—such as those conducted by Rand Corporation and The Dartmouth Atlas—have provided ample evidence of the unexplained geographic variation in the style, delivery, and cost of healthcare. Second, the unsustainable rise in healthcare expenditures has forced employers, third-party payers, and government payers to seek methods of ensuring appropriate and cost-effective delivery of care. Third, the introduction of the Medicare Spending Per Beneficiary efficiency indicator, which has been used since 2015 to levy penalties against hospitals, has increased attention on the appropriate use of therapeutic interventions. Fourth, the Merit-based Incentive Payment System payment methodology includes a resource component that will affect how physicians get paid. Fifth, the steady move toward a value-based healthcare system, an evolution expedited by new regulations, new payment models, and promulgated by commercial as well as government payers, has set the stage for new payment models that expect lower costs across the continuum and better patient quality outcomes. It is the anticipation of these value payment models and the expectation of care coordination across the continuum that are the primary drivers of cost reductions and will supersede the age-old call to "reduce the length of stay!"

Many medical societies and professional organizations publish medical guidelines that are primarily derived from a comprehensive and systematic review of published research studies. Despite some physicians' protests that this amounts to "cookbook medicine," the medical field is constantly evolving, with new research findings and best practices continuously becoming available. Protocols enable the medical staff to question the value of traditional diagnostic tests and practice patterns in light of new research. Hospital medical staff use them to develop community-specific clinical protocols that reflect current practice and can be translated into a standardized medical treatment plan for key diagnoses to improve routine treatment and clinical outcomes for hospitalized patients.

It is often said that half of what physicians learn in medical school is either incorrect or becomes obsolete, but it is impossible to know what half. It is therefore incumbent on physicians to continue their education—learning about new treatments and medications through journals, grand rounds, and continuing medical education programs. Although continuing medical education is required to maintain licensure, the main motivation for physicians should be to ensure they are providing their patients the best care possible based on the most recent findings. The payers devote extensive resources to ensure that enrollees receive the best medical care available in the most cost-effective setting. Professional societies such as the American College of Physicians and quasi-government agencies such as the National Quality Forum develop practice guidelines that quickly become recognized as the standard of care and are subsequently adopted by payers. These guidelines are subject to extensive peer review and then published for use by all medical professionals and collated by the government at *www.guidelines.gov*. Many payers have also published their coverage guidelines online for use by patients, physicians, and UR specialists. It falls on everyone to ensure that every patient receives the right care in the right setting.

The key for any progressive hospital medical staff is to stay at the forefront of medical knowledge and determine which interventions can truly help patients. However, protocols are not set in stone—that's why they are often referred to as practice guidelines. They provide physicians and clinicians with recommendations for best practice in the diagnosis and treatment of specific and more frequently encountered conditions to optimize patient care. As the evidence changes, so should the protocol. A protocol does not have to be used if any part of it is not appropriate for a particular patient with a specific condition, but documentation should support variation from the protocol.

The use of social media has also grown exponentially in all facets of life, including medicine. This has meant that physicians and other healthcare providers can interact with colleagues not only in their hospital but around the world. While in the past a notable article would appear in a medical journal, possibly accompanied by an editorial written by a key opinion leader from that specialty, and a practicing physician would need to find the time to read and assimilate the information, now a new article or study presented at a conference can lead to a discussion among hundreds, providing that physician many views and expert interpretations of the issue.

Nothing demonstrates this more than the spread of medical information, and misinformation, on social media during the COVID-19 pandemic. At the onset of the pandemic, there were many online discussions about the difficulty of adequately ventilating patients with acute respiratory failure with a high mortality rate and whether this represents typical acute respiratory distress syndrome. Discussions of anecdotes on Twitter among critical care physicians led to the realization that patients with COVID-19 can tolerate markedly low oxygen levels if placed in the prone position. These discussions spread quickly and led to the adoption of a unique way of treating acute respiratory failure from COVID-19, saving the lives of countless patients. At the same time, misinformation spread about various drug therapies, including hydroxychloroquine and ivermectin, and the safety and efficacy of the COVID-19 vaccine led to patients avoiding medical care and self-treating with unknown consequences.

Choosing wisely

In a special communication from *JAMA* in 2019 that prompted many responses from other medical journals, as well as the lay press, researchers cited that overtreatment or low-value medical interventions cost upwards of $101.2 billion. The researchers used 54 different publications that included information on six areas previously identified by the National Institute of Medicine as important in quantifying waste: failure of care delivery, failure of care coordination, overtreatment or low-value care, overpricing of treatments and medication, fraud and abuse, and administrative complexity. Taken together, waste in healthcare could be costing as much as $935 billion annually, according to the researchers' conclusions (Shrank, 2019).

In an effort to combat waste due to overtreatment or low value, the American Board of Internal Medicine created the Choosing Wisely® initiative to promote conversations between patients and providers about the use and overuse of tests and procedures that are often unnecessary, drive up costs, and could put patients at risk. The campaign provides a list of medical interventions that physicians should not provide for their patients. For example, the list for hospitalists includes items such as, "don't order continuous telemetry monitoring outside of the ICU without using a protocol that governs continuation," or "don't place, or leave in place, urinary catheters for incontinence or convenience or monitoring of output for non-critically ill patients" (Society of Hospital Medicine—Adult Hospital Medicine, 2013). New York's Mount Sinai Hospital launched a "Lose the Tube" study based on this standard and reduced urinary tract infection rates from 2.85 to 0.32 per 1,000 catheter days and reduced costs by $32,245 (Cho et al., 2017).

Contrary to popular perception, programs striving for best practice do not focus on simply reducing utilization. Rather, the goal is to reduce inappropriate use of medical interventions, which includes not only overuse but also misuse and underuse. The UR committee serves as a forum to motivate the medical staff to adopt and implement evidence-based guidelines. These guidelines can also be excellent tools for the case manager and UR specialist to monitor the patient's progression of care. They represent a proven mechanism for promoting cost-conscious, appropriate care and for identifying interventions that add questionable value to the care of the patient. Access to medical staff–approved guidelines and related order sets represents a best practice feature in highly successful organizations.

While many physicians view order sets as another element of "cookbook medicine," the reality is that no one physician can remember every detail every time. Many physicians use mnemonics to try to recall all the items required when ordering admission (e.g., ADCVANDISSL: admit, diagnosis, condition, vitals, activity, nursing, diet, intake and outpatient, specific medications, symptomatic medications, labs). But imagine the patient admitted with a stroke where the physician forgets to order a speech therapy evaluation. That patient will have a longer-than-necessary period without oral intake until it is realized that speech therapy was not ordered and the provider can be contacted to see the patient and assess their swallowing. A stroke order set, based on evidence-based protocols, which includes orders for speech therapy, and much more, would prevent such an occurrence. The use of order sets in such situations is a form of cognitive offloading. In simple terms, it takes away the "thinking" needed to remember the mundane things, like ordering therapy, so the physician can concentrate on the things that do require thinking, such as determining the cause of the stroke and deciding on the best treatment.

The 2-midnight rule

Once medical necessity is confirmed, the next necessary decision is whether to place the patient in outpatient with observation or admit the patient as inpatient based on the expectation of two midnights of medically necessary hospital care. Although some medical literature may report average LOS for a limited number of diseases, and some of the screening tools report on optimal LOS, the decision is usually based on clinical judgment and experience. CMS states the following:

> *The decision to admit a patient as an inpatient is a complex medical decision based on many factors, including the risk of an adverse event during the period considered for hospitalization, and an assessment of the services that the beneficiary will need during the hospital stay.* (CMS, 2017)

On August 19, 2013, CMS published the 2014 IPPS final rule, which included a section establishing the 2-midnight rule as the basis for admission decisions. Prior to this rule, the physician decided to admit a patient as inpatient based on the perceived risk of not doing so, as well as an anticipated LOS of more than 24 hours. Because of ambiguities in determining risk and weak documentation, auditors subsequently denied many of these admissions, resulting in a large backlog of appeals.

To attempt to alleviate this backlog and establish a reasonable admission standard, CMS developed the 2-midnight rule, which removed risk from the decision and states that a physician should admit a patient as inpatient if he or she determines that the patient requires hospital care and the LOS is expected to extend over two midnights. As will be discussed later, in 2016 CMS did reinsert risk as a factor in the determination. CMS clarified that its previous 24-hour benchmark is still pertinent, but this new stipulation reflects the 24-hour period between two midnights, which CMS refers to as a Medicare utilization day. The use of midnights also allows CMS and its contactors to use the information that is already found on the UB-04 claim (the form that the federal government and commercial payers use to submit hospital claims) to determine whether the stay exceeded one Medicare utilization day (two midnights), rather than requiring the hospital to report the time at which care began and ended on the UB-04.

The first step in the application of the 2-midnight rule is the decision to hospitalize a patient. In the 2014 IPPS final rule, CMS states, "The crux of the medical decision is the choice to keep the beneficiary at the hospital in order to receive services or reduce risk, or discharge the beneficiary home because they may be safely treated through intermittent outpatient visits or some other care." This means that patients who require hospital care should be hospitalized, but those who can safely be treated at home or in a setting less intense than a hospital do not require hospital care and should not be hospitalized. CMS expects physicians with the guidance of the ARS to make this decision independent of cost or availability of resources.

For example, if an elderly patient who lives alone is brought to the hospital because he or she is falling and cannot safely live alone and it is determined there are no acute injuries or acute decompensation of any medical conditions, then the patient does not require hospitalization. He or she can be safely cared for at home with a home aide or could securely reside in a nursing facility. Such a patient typically does not require services that can only be provided in a hospital, nor is this patient at short-term medical risk that requires him or her to be monitored in the hospital.

Similarly, consider the patient who states that he or she is unable to afford an antibiotic for a simple urinary tract infection. The patient should not be hospitalized for administration of intravenous antibiotics. Instead, the UR specialist or social worker should work with the patient to find a payer source or a less expensive medication, because he or she can safely be treated with oral antibiotics outside of a hospital.

Although the decision about the need for hospitalization is usually straightforward, there are occasional circumstances in which a patient who does not require hospitalization must be hospitalized because there is no safe discharge plan. Because lack of a safe discharge plan does not constitute medical necessity for hospital care, hospitals cannot charge Medicare or commercial insurers for such care; it is considered the hospital's social service mission to the community to care for such patients until a safe discharge can be arranged. These patients should be hospitalized as outpatients rather than admitted as inpatients. The nuances of billing for their care are beyond the scope of this text.

Once it is established that the patient requires hospital care as defined by CMS, the ARS—in collaboration with the admitting physician—must then determine whether the patient's care is expected to surpass two midnights. An inpatient admission begins on the calendar date that the admission order is written, but the 2-midnight clock begins at the exact time that the patient begins receiving care in the hospital, excluding triage services.

For example, if a patient presents with abdominal pain and the triage nurse obtains vital signs and then orders a complete blood count and chemistry panel based on the department's protocol for abdominal pain, the time that the nurse ordered the blood tests would start the midnight clock. This differentiation between the inpatient clock and the 2-midnight clock is important for the patient presenting close to midnight, as a patient whose care begins almost at midnight would pass his or her first midnight relatively quickly, whereas one whose care does not begin until just after midnight would not pass his or her first midnight for almost 24 hours.

CMS also expects care that is provided efficiently and without delay for hospital, doctor, or patient convenience. With some exceptions, CMS expects patients with common "rule-out" diagnoses, such as abdominal pain, syncope, and TIA, to be evaluated and released prior to the passing of two midnights. Inpatient admission is appropriate if the evaluation, which is often done in a clinical decision unit (observational care), reveals an abnormality that requires additional care that can only be safely provided in the hospital setting, or if the patient continues to require medically necessary services that can only safely be provided in the hospital and that care will pass the second midnight.

Determination of proper status

For patients with fee-for-service Medicare, the proper status can be determined using the same two-step process. First, ask whether the patient requires hospital care, and then estimate how many midnights that hospital care is expected to pass. If more than two midnights are expected and supported by documentation in the medical record, then the patient should be admitted as an inpatient. Many commercial insurers, MA insurers, and Medicaid plans continue to differentiate between inpatient and outpatient status based on the intensity of service, severity of illness, or the use of other proprietary rules and guidelines independent of the two-midnight time element adopted by Medicare. If this is encountered at your hospital, consider the circumstances at the next contract renewal negotiations.

Because of these varying definitions of status and level of care used by Medicare and commercial insurers, work with the registration staff to ensure that the demographic information is updated and accurate so that the correct guidelines can be used. If the insurer requires concurrent notification of admissions and review of criteria, ensure that the correct criteria set is used and that the two-step process is completed. This process includes a first-level criteria and documentation review by the ARS, followed by a second-level review by a PA if first-level criteria are not met and the admitting physician is reluctant to modify his or her documentation. The complete information is then conveyed to the insurer. If the insurer will not authorize the admission based on secondary review, request a peer-to-peer review with the plan medical director and your PA or attending physician.

2-midnight benchmark admissions

It is not unusual for patients to receive treatment spanning at least one midnight while still an outpatient, either in the ED, operating room, recovery room, or a clinical decision unit (area designated for outpatient/ observation patients). If it is determined that they require more care to either reduce risk or to receive services that can only be provided in the hospital and the total time will pass the second midnight, then the rule specifies that the patient should be admitted as inpatient—even if the patient goes home the next day (before three midnights pass).

CMS refers to this as a "benchmark" admission in that the total length of hospital care has exceeded its benchmark of two midnights. The key determinant here is the medical necessity of continued hospital care as opposed to continued hospitalization as a convenience to the hospital, physician, or patient. Clearly, a patient that is stable for discharge at 6 p.m. but unwilling to drive home in the dark does not require hospital care and should not be admitted as an inpatient. However, a patient with asthma who was treated over one midnight as an outpatient with observation and continues to require frequent nebulizer treatments and intravenous steroids should be admitted as an inpatient prior to the second midnight.

The physician should document the justification for continuing hospitalization in the medical record, including response to treatment, indications for continued treatment, and plans for care. The notes by the patient's nurse and any ancillary caregivers (e.g., respiratory therapists) and the ongoing assessments and responses to treatment are equally important but less scrutinized. When completely documented, the information allows the auditors and other caregivers to understand the severity of the patient's illness and justifies the need for continuing care in the hospital. Once again, the narrative portion of such documentation is crucial; documentation consisting of a series of checked boxes cannot adequately paint this picture, especially if the checked boxes directly contradict information in the narrative notes.

It should also be noted that the determination of medical necessity for continuing hospitalization should follow the same guidelines as the initial decision to hospitalize the patient. In other words, could the patient be discharged and safely treated in a lesser setting? Commercial criteria can assist the UR staff in making this determination in that if the patient passes criteria at any level, it denotes that hospital care is necessary and inpatient admission should be ordered. But if criteria are not met, a secondary review should be performed. A simple way to think about this question is to ask whether the patient could be discharged and see their physician in the office the next day or must they stay in the hospital for treatment or monitoring.

When discussing use of the 2-midnight rule, also consider postoperative care of a patient who underwent outpatient surgery. The payment to the hospital for an outpatient surgery includes all necessary hospital care for routine recovery. Once that period ends, if it is determined and documented appropriately that the patient will require hospitalization that will pass the second midnight, then the physician should admit the patient as an inpatient. For instance, the normal recovery after transurethral resection of the prostate often includes one night in the hospital for bladder irrigation. If, because of the presence of persistent hematuria, the urologist on the first postoperative day determines that the patient requires a second midnight in the hospital for bladder irrigation and monitoring, then the patient should be admitted as an inpatient, and the physician should complete the supporting documentation in the medical record. The same standard applies as above: can the patient be discharged home and safely receive care? In this example, continuous bladder irrigation cannot be safely provided in any other setting, and a patient who continues to bleed warrants ongoing monitoring in a hospital.

Transfer patients and the 2-midnight rule

The 2-midnight rule changes the way that status determinations for patient transfers are handled. If a patient needs hospital care that is expected to require more than two midnights but the plan at the time of admission to the originating hospital is to transfer the patient to another facility prior to the second midnight, then he or she should be placed as outpatient with observation services at the originating hospital. If the patient requires hospital care at the originating hospital that is expected to exceed two midnights and the initial plan is to care for the patient at the original hospital but transfer the patient if his or her condition deteriorates, then the patient should be admitted as an inpatient. If the patient is subsequently transferred, even within hours of admission, the billing status remains inpatient based on the initial plan. The crucial factor here is the expectation of the time the patient will remain at the hospital as of the time of the admission decision, after the emergency department evaluation.

The ARS in access management at the receiving hospitals should now consider any medically necessary midnights spent at the transferring hospital (including time spent in the ED at the sending hospital) and the number of anticipated midnights at their institution when deciding on the proper status. For example, if a patient spent two or more midnights at the originating hospital and is transferred for a procedure that may not require another midnight (i.e., a cardiac catheterization after a myocardial infarction), then the UR specialist at the receiving hospital should still recommend inpatient admission. The stay at the receiving hospital may not pass any midnights, but the rule states the receiving hospital should admit the patient as inpatient. The patient will incur an inpatient deductible for the admission at the first hospital, but because the admission to the second hospital is within the 60-day "spell of illness," there is no deductible for that second admission. Payment to the receiving hospital will be based on the Medicare Severity Diagnosis-Related Group (MS-DRG) to which the patient's admission is coded, and the payment to the sending hospital, if they were admitted as inpatient, will depend on the coded DRG, the number of days the patient remained at that hospital, and the geometric mean length of stay for that DRG. It will also not be considered a readmission as part of CMS' Hospital Readmission Reduction Program, as the index admission will be coded using discharge status 02 (transfer to another acute care hospital), which is not counted as a readmission. CMS has allowed hospitals to place occurrence span code 72 on the claim of a patient who did not spend two inpatient midnights at the hospital but whose total medically necessary care at that hospital or another hospital exceeded two midnights. The code will alert the Medicare contactors that the 2-midnight benchmark was met.

Exceptions to the 2-midnight rule

Medicare has also indicated several exceptions to the 2-midnight rule. The first is that patients admitted for inpatient-only surgeries—which must be performed as inpatient—do not have to spend two midnights in the hospital. The surgeon may discharge the patient whenever doing so is clinically appropriate, including on the day of surgery. CMS has specified that if an inpatient is discharged prior to the passing of one midnight, a bed charge may be added to the claim to avoid any potential edits. In no circumstance should a physician be told that they must keep a patient overnight simply to accrue a night in the hospital as inpatient.

Another exception are patients who require unanticipated mechanical ventilation but are expected to require less than two midnights of hospital care. Such situations most commonly occur with patients experiencing drug overdose or intoxication and who require intubation and mechanical ventilation for airway protection until they wake up. This could also apply to the patient who had an outpatient surgery with general anesthesia but who upon extubation is unable to maintain his or her oxygenation and requires reintubation for a limited period of time until the anesthetic wears off. Note that this exception would not apply to that same patient if he or she was unable to be extubated in the recovery room and must continue mechanical ventilation until he or she is able to be extubated. In this case, mechanical ventilation is expected as part of the surgery, and the inability to extubate would not warrant inpatient admission unless and until the patient's care is expected to pass the second midnight.

In January 2016, as part of the 2016 OPPS final rule and in response to stakeholder feedback, CMS added a third exception to the 2-midnight rule. CMS stated that they will allow for Medicare Part A payment on a *case-by-case* basis for inpatient admissions that do not satisfy the 2-midnight benchmark if the documentation in the medical record supports the admitting physician's determination that the patient requires inpatient hospital care despite an expected LOS that is less than two midnights. Physicians should make this determination using the severity of the signs and symptoms exhibited by the patient, the medical predictability of something adverse happening to the patient, and the risk.

There was a lot of confusion when this new exception was first announced, as severity of signs and symptoms was a factor that physicians used prior to the 2-midnight rule and that led to the large number of denials. After a period of uncertainty, one of the QIOs indicated that this exception could apply to patients who presented with life-threatening illnesses that could be rapidly treated and that frequently resolve within one day, such as acute myocardial infarctions, diabetic ketoacidosis, stroke with successful administration of thrombolytic therapy in the ED, and hyperkalemia with electrocardiographic changes in a dialysis patient. As noted above, this exception can also be used for patients who are hospitalized for surgery. Those who have a one-midnight expectation but are at high risk of an adverse event may be admitted as inpatient if that risk is delineated in the medical record and the admission order is written preoperatively.

Inpatients who spend fewer than two midnights in the hospital

There will also be a subset of patients who are admitted as inpatient based on the expectation of a 2-midnight hospitalization but who are subsequently discharged prior to the second midnight. These patients are not exceptions to the 2-midnight rule—they meet the rule by virtue of the expectation of a 2-midnight-or-greater stay at the time of the admission decision, but it turns out that they did not pass that second midnight. If formally admitted with an inpatient order from a qualified practitioner, these admissions may be compliantly billed as an inpatient admission.

Such admissions include patients who die prior to the second midnight and those who are admitted but subsequently leave the hospital against medical advice (AMA). In the case of an AMA discharge, if there is documentation that the physician recommends continuing medically necessary hospital care but the patient chooses to assume the risks and leave the hospital, then the admission may be billed as inpatient. It should be noted that a signed "Against Medical Advice" form is not a regulatory requirement; the physician may discharge the patient in a collegial manner with prescriptions and discharge instructions, as long as there is proper documentation of the discussion and of risks to the patient.

Hospice exceptions

Patients who elect to receive hospice care after inpatient admission and are subsequently transferred to hospice in the hospital or another setting or home represent another subset of those who meet the 2-midnight rule without staying for two midnights. In this case, the decision to elect hospice must occur after formal admission. A patient who elects hospice care in the ED prior to admission would not be admitted as inpatient. Instead, he or she could be placed as outpatient with observation if acute care is needed for symptom control and/or to arrange hospice placement.

Rapid recovery

The last subset of patients who meet the 2-midnight expectation are patients who have an unexpectedly rapid recovery. If a patient is appropriately admitted as inpatient based on an expectation of a 2-midnight stay but improves more quickly than expected, then the patient can be discharged prior to the second midnight, and the admission can be billed as inpatient. In this case, the medical record will be reviewed for evidence that the admission decision was correct and that there is documentation that the patient improved faster than expected.

For example, if a patient presents with a mild exacerbation of heart failure with normal vital signs, no hypoxia, and only mild edema and is admitted as inpatient and discharged the next day after diuresing 1,000 cc of urine, then the decision to admit as an inpatient will be questioned. However, consider the patient who was tachycardic and hypoxic and was expected to need three to four days in the hospital for diuresis and medication adjustment but then diuresed 4,000 cc with two doses of diuretics, felt dramatically better the next day, and was discharged. In this instance, the admission decision was correct, and the patient can be seen as having an unexpectedly rapid recovery. The physician should document a phrase such as "the patient improved faster than expected" in a progress note or the discharge summary to emphasize that the patient was initially expected to require hospital care over two midnights (even though this could be inferred from the documentation). The physician could also incorporate this unexpectedly rapid recovery as an addendum to the medical record, following conventional rules for adding documentation to a hospital chart after discharge.

Because these short inpatient admissions are likely to be audited, all zero- and one-day inpatient admissions should be reviewed by the audit team. In larger hospitals, audit teams are typically part of the office of the chief compliance officer, whereas in smaller hospitals, they may live within the revenue cycle under finance or within the UR department. Prebilling audits ensure that the case fits either an exception or an acceptable case and that the documentation supports that. If the documentation is not adequate, then the physician should be asked to add an addendum to the medical record providing further information. If it is determined that the original admission decision was not correct, the self-denial and Part B rebilling processes should be followed. This process requires involvement of the physician members of the UR committee.

Observation services

Successful observation models include a dedicated unit design, known most often as clinical decision units (CDU), with dedicated beds and specialized staff. Well-managed CDUs optimize inpatient and ED flow, increase acute capacity, improve patient satisfaction, and ultimately maintain a higher level of quality patient care. Scattered bed models, where outpatients are integrated into the acute care environment, challenge medical and nursing resources and are inefficient, confusing the patients and their families, and lack specific protocols, which often results in stays greater than 24 hours.

CMS defines observation as follows:

> A well-defined set of specific, clinically appropriate services, which include ongoing short-term treatment, assessment, and reassessment before a decision can be made regarding whether patients will require further treatment as hospital inpatients or if they are able to be discharged from the hospital. (CMS, 2015a)

As can be seen from that definition, observation is a hospital service used to decide whether a patient needs to be admitted as an inpatient. Observation is often characterized as a seamless extension of the information-gathering and decision-making process used in the emergency department (ED). Although Medicare limits coverage of observation services to 48 hours by way of the 2-midnight rule, the National Correct Coding Initiative has an edit that kicks in at 72 hours. Medicare pays hospitals a comprehensive Ambulatory Payment Classification (C-APC) rate (C-APC 8011) by bundling all the services provided during observation, including room and board, nursing services, labs, and imaging. Payment method by commercial insurance companies is determined contractually. Observation stays of less than 24 hours have traditionally been a hospital benchmark since they give physician enough time to determine whether the patient's underlying clinical condition justified inpatient admission, but by no means should this be considered "a line in the sand." For example, the patient who presents to the ED at 1 a.m. with dyspnea and is placed outpatient with observation at 3 a.m. would reach the 24-hour mark at 3 a.m. the next day but would not reach the two midnight mark until 45 hours after the start of observation. There must be a physician order for observation services in order to bill for it.

If there is a question as to whether the patient will require two midnights of care or does not fit into one of the exceptions to the two-midnight expectation, then the patient should be placed as an outpatient with observation services. However, observation should not be a catch-all category to provide services, nor should it be a strategy to decompress ED crowding, which is not, unfortunately, uncommon. Headlines about the financial consequence of outpatient/observation misuse raise the ire of the community and have generated several lawsuits, one of which resulted in the creation of the Medicare Outpatient Observation Notice form (MOON) and, in 2020, another which gave Medicare beneficiaries the right to appeal a retrospective change in status from inpatient to outpatient. This 2020 case is interesting because of the judge's "frustration with the inpatient-outpatient industrial complex." Attorney Judy Waltz noted that "patient status as inpatient or observation is an artificial distinction" that has no effect on patient care and exists solely for payment purposes. "The determination of patient status is made by physicians who have no financial skin in the game and by hospital utilization review committees that try to get it right" (Youngstrom, 2020). This decision is being appealed by CMS, and as of this writing there are no formal appeal rights available to the patient whose status is changed to outpatient.

Finally, physicians should not order observation for care that is normally included in the payment for a provided service, such as for routine recovery after an outpatient surgery or procedure or prior to the completion of the ED evaluation. For example, the normal recovery period for an outpatient surgery is defined by what that particular physician considers the normal recovery period. A simple surgery such as an incision and drainage may have a routine recovery of 30 minutes, a hernia repair may have a routine recovery of four to six hours, and a simple mastectomy may have a routine recovery that continues until the day after surgery. It is only when routine recovery ends that the physician may order observation. Unfortunately, many commercial insurers will authorize an overnight stay after an outpatient surgery by approving "an observation stay," confusing physicians and UR staff as to the proper application of the rule.

References

Cho, H. J., et al. (1 March 2017). "Lose the Tube": A Choosing Wisely initiative to reduce catheter-associated urinary tract infections in hospitalist-led inpatient units. *American Journal of Infection Control, 45*(3): 333–335.

Centers for Medicare & Medicaid Services. (CMS). (19 August 2013). FY 2014 Inpatient Prospective Payment System Final Rule. *Federal Register, 78*(160)50944. Retrieved from *https://www.gpo.gov/fdsys/pkg/FR-2013-08-19/html/2013-18956.htm.*

CMS. (12 March 2014). Reviewing Hospital Claims for Patient Status: Admissions On or After October 1, 2013. Retrieved from *https://www.cms.gov/Research-Statistics-Data-and-Systems/Monitoring-Programs/Medicare-FFS-Compliance-Programs/Medical-Review/Downloads/ReviewingHospitalClaimsforAdmissionforPosting03122014.pdf.*

CMS. (2015a). Chapter 6: Hospital Services Covered Under Part B. *Medicare Benefit Policy Manual.* Retrieved from *https://www.cms.gov/Regulations-and-Guidance/Guidance/Manuals/downloads/bp102c06.pdf.*

CMS. (2015b). Medicare Claims Processing Transmittal 3238: April 2015 Update of the Hospital Outpatient Prospective Payment System. Retrieved from *https://www.cms.gov/Regulations-and-Guidance/Guidance/Transmittals/Downloads/R3238CP.pdf.*

CMS. (2017). Chapter 1: Inpatient Hospital Services Covered Under Part A. *Medicare Benefit Policy Manual.* Retrieved from *https://www.cms.gov/Regulations-and-Guidance/Guidance/Manuals/downloads/bp102c01.pdf.*

CMS. (14 December 2017). Hospital Outpatient Prospective Payment and Ambulatory Surgical Center Payment Systems and Quality Reporting Programs Final Rule. *Federal Register, 82*(239):59384. Retrieved from *https://www.gpo.gov/fdsys/pkg/FR-2017-12-14/pdf/R1-2017-23932.pdf.*

CMS. (December 2020) Medicare Program: Hospital Outpatient Prospective Payment and Ambulatory Surgical Center Payment Systems and Quality Reporting Programs. Retrieved from https://www.cms.gov/Medicare/Medicare-Fee-for-Service-Payment/ASCPayment/ASC-Regulations-and-Notices-Items/CMS-1717-FC.

CMS. (18 May 2021). Medicare Program; Medicare Coverage of Innovative Technology (MCIT) and Definition of "Reasonable and Necessary"; Delay of Effective Date. Retrieved from *https://www.federalregister.gov/documents/2021/05/18/2021-10466/medicare-program-medicare-coverage-of-innovative-technology-mcit-and-definition-of-reasonable-and.*

CMS. (19 July 2021). Medicare Program: Hospital Outpatient Prospective Payment and Ambulatory Surgical Center Payment Systems and Quality Reporting Programs; Price Transparency of Hospital Standard Charges; Radiation Oncology Model; Request for Information on Rural Emergency Hospitals. Page 347:IX(B). Retrieved from *https://public-inspection.federalregister.gov/2021-15496.pdf.*

Hirsch, R. (2018). Inpatient admission order regulations continue to confound. RAC Monitor. Retrieved from *https://racmonitor.com/inpatient-admission-order-regulations-continue-to-confound/*.

Shrank, W. H., Rogstad, T. L., Parekh, N. (2019). Waste in the US Health Care System. *JAMA, 322*(15): 1501–1509. doi:10.1001/jama.2019.13978.

Tajirian, T., Stergiopoulos, V., Strudwick, G., Sequeira, L., Sanches, M., Kemp, J., Ramamoorthi, K., Zhang, T., and Jankowicz, D. (1 July 2020). The Influence of Electronic Health Record Use on Physician Burnout: Cross-Sectional Survey. *Journal of Medical Internet Research 22*(7). Retrieved from *https://www.jmir.org/2020/7/e19274*.

Wang, M. D., Khanna, R., Najafi, N. (2017). Characterizing the source of text in electronic health record program notes. *JAMA Internal Medicine, 177*(8):1212–1213. doi:10.1001/jamainternmed.2017.1548.

Youngstrom, N. (30 March 2020). Court says inpatients changed to observation have right to appeal, orders new process. Retrieved from *https://www.jdsupra.com/legalnews/court-says-inpatients-changed-to-70053/*.

CHAPTER 6

The Utilization Review Process: Continued-Stay and Post-Acute Activities

Continued-Stay Review

Utilization review (UR) specialists speak a different language than most other hospital associates, and nowhere is it more apparent than in discussing a patient's need for continued stay with the patient's physician. Physicians are not schooled in regulatory requirements nor the economic dynamics associated with medical necessity, and many, especially those who receive fee-for-service payment for services, are not incentivized to explain the rationale or give evidence to support the patient's continued stay in the hospital. Nevertheless, the rules of medical necessity continue to apply to patients during the entirety of their hospitalization, and utilization management (UM) remains the primary approach that public and private payers use to determine if patients are receiving appropriate care and if the money spent on healthcare is providing value.

The rules governing Medicare are pretty explicit when it comes to determining medical necessity at the time of admission. But, with the exception of the requirements for outlier certification at the 20th day, there is nothing in the regulations that dictates continued-stay review schedules. The timing of Medicare continued-stay reviews is whatever is stated in the hospital's plan. This is a key requirement. If the hospitals plan states that Medicare reviews are to be done every other day, that will be the standard against which the hospital will be evaluated during accreditation processes. That is why we strongly suggest that the UR plan should avoid specific processes and instead rely on the use of policies and procedures, which are more easily modified.

The *Interpretive Guidelines for CoP* §482.30(d) address the issue of the medical necessity for continued stay and spells out the process to intervene. The process is almost exactly like that for condition code (CC44): one UR committee physician can make the determination that continued stay is not necessary if the attending physician concurs, or if the "attending practitioner does not respond or does not contest the findings of the committee or subgroup or those of the physician who performed the initial review, then the findings are final." Two UR committee physicians are needed if the attending physician disagrees. In either case, "notification must be given, no later than 2 days after the determination, to the hospital, the patient (or next of kin), the practitioners or practitioners responsible for the care of the patient, and the hospital administrator" (CMS, 2020). The state also must be notified in the case of Medicaid.

Every patient should have an admission review at the point of entry and, if done routinely and rigorously, the next review for Medicare patients can be scheduled for the trim point—the geometric mean length of stay (GMLOS) assigned to the working diagnosis-related group (DRG) based on the patient's primary diagnosis and any secondary diagnoses. Note that the GMLOS is not the same as the average length of stay (ALOS). The ALOS equals the sum of all LOSs divided by the number of stays. For example, two stays, one that is four days and one that is 12 days, equal a total of 16 days, which divided by two equals an ALOS of eight days. But GMLOS multiplies the lengths of stay and then computes the square root of the product (48), which is 6.928 days. In this manner, the statistical impact of outliers is lessened.

Medicare is not as stringent as commercial payers when it comes to reviewing every day of a beneficiary's hospitalization and, as long as the patient continues to receive care that cannot be safely provided at a lower level of care, a formal review is generally not necessary. As cited in the *CoP*, "hospitals need review only cases that they reasonably assume to be outlier cases based on extended length of stay, as described in § 412.80(a)(1)(i)." Medicare's concern is that a continued stay after the point at which outlier status is reached will result in a higher payment to the hospital, and it wants to be sure the stay remains medically necessary to justify the extra payment. Given the overwhelming continued-stay reviews demanded by Medicare Advantage (MA) payers, Medicare's standard should be considered when determining the best way to assess continued stay among regular Medicare patients. On the other hand, because most hospital stays are paid as a fixed DRG payment, it is in the hospital's best financial interest to ensure that the length of stay is only as long as medically necessary and cost per case does not exceed DRG payment. To better understand this premise, consider Dr. A's patient with a LOS of five days and less costs than anticipated payment. Then consider Dr. B's patient with a LOS of four days and more costs than anticipated payment. If throughput is the primary hospital concern, then Dr. B's management of her patient is highly desirable. But if margin is the primary hospital goal, then Dr. A's patient care management is highly favorable. Regular reviews and access to the relevant information to consider these issues can detect that inflection point and can help the hospital maintain its operating margin.

One of the advantages of assigning UR specialists to groups of physicians (e.g., hospitalists) or by specific payers is that it gives the UR specialists the opportunity to becomes familiar with the same group of patients under the physicians' care and can estimate anticipated discharge and help the hospitalist document accordingly. It also gives the UR specialists the opportunity to learn how each hospitalist provides care. Admittedly, this suggestion works best if the UR specialists are on the patient unit, participate in rounds, speak to the nurses and hospitalists, and can observe patients. Today, with continued-stay reviews often being done electronically from a reviewer's home or a centralized corporate office, it is more of a challenge.

Continued-stay reviews for commercial patients are another story entirely. For these patients, review obligations are established in the contract or provider manual. If your contract or provider manual does not address this, then the UR specialist must jump to the payer's demands. Allowing the payers to call at whim whenever they need a piece of information is disruptive and can be overwhelming and should be addressed during contract negotiation. A Health Insurance Portability and Accountability Act of 1996 (HIPAA)-compliant portal into the hospital's electronic health record (EHR) should be considered. If this option is used, the hospital should protect itself by ensuring the contract addendum addresses notification following the payer's electronic review. Once again, the way the payer compensates the hospital for inpatient admissions, with a DRG model, a per diem rate, or a percent of charges, often determines how often the payer will perform reviews and how often a hospital should perform reviews themselves. In turn, this emphasizes the need for accurate patient registration information.

Condition code 44: Correcting incorrect inpatient admission status

If a hospital has a robust, seven-day access management program in place, every inpatient will have documentation supporting their need for inpatient care. However, there are times when a Medicare patient is admitted but subsequent review fails to adequately demonstrate the necessity for inpatient admission. There are two options for correcting these situations, the first being the use of the condition code 44 (CC44) process while the patient is still hospitalized. The second is the self-denial and rebill process, which will be discussed later in this chapter.

In discussing CC44, keep the following three things in mind. One, the process was intended to be used occasionally, not as a substitute for an assertive medical necessity review at the time of admission. Overuse of CC44 is a red flag to MACs. Two, a UR committee physician must be involved. Even the physician who wrote the original admission order may not unilaterally revert the patient's status from inpatient to outpatient with a few keystrokes. And three, the hospital may not use an outsourced physician advisor service to authorize a CC44 change on a Medicare patient. The UR committee physician member must be a voting member of the hospital's medical staff.

It should also be noted that many MA payers require the use of CC44. This is an area of great misunderstanding by even the most seasoned UR specialists and physician advisors (Ugarte Hopkins, 2021). First, requiring CC44 is not the same as requiring the Medicare CC44 *process*. Remember that a condition code is simply a number that must be placed on a claim when a specific circumstance occurs. In the case of CC44, it is required when a patient's status has changed from inpatient to outpatient. In many cases, a MA plan patient has been formally admitted as inpatient but the MA plan will not authorize inpatient admission. If the hospital agrees that inpatient admission was inappropriate, the hospital can simply obtain a new order from the physician and change the patient's status to outpatient. (The option to object to the change and fight this with a peer-to-peer discussion or appeal is also available.) In this circumstance, review by a physician member of the UR committee is not necessary. Then, if the plan "requires CC44," the UR specialist can simply notify the billing staff to ensure that "44" gets entered in the proper form locator on the UB-04 or the electronic equivalent. The CC44 process, on the other hand, is reserved for situations where internal review by the hospital and the UR committee physician determines that inpatient admission was not necessary. This distinction is important, because the CC44 process requires much more work than simply adding a "44" to the claim.

The start of any day for a UR specialist begins with the review of patients who were admitted without benefit of an admission review, admitted with questionable documentation, or placed in observation. An admission that falls into the first or second category is a priority since the clock starts ticking on the remedy to resolve. Following review of the documentation and guidelines related to the physician's preliminary diagnosis, the UR specialist will check on the current condition of the patient and may get in contact with the physician to seek clarification, if required, of medical necessity. If clarification is not forthcoming, then the UR specialist will contact the physician advisor or a physician member of the UR committee to review the case. If the physician determines that the inpatient admission was not appropriate, then the attending physician must be contacted and given the opportunity to provide input. If the attending agrees, an order should be obtained from the attending to change the patient's status to outpatient. At that point, written notification must be provided to the patient, the physician, and the hospital within two days, but preferably at the time of the change. If all criteria for changing status from inpatient to outpatient are met:

1. Bill the entire episode as though the inpatient admission never occurred

2. Use bill type 13X or 85X

3. Cite CC44 on the claim form in one of the Form Locators 24–30

4. Include charges for services that were furnished per a physician order

At the time the status is changed to outpatient, an order for observation services can be obtained if the patient requires continued care in the hospital. Only observation services that are provided after this order can be placed on the claim. The hours that preceded the change are not billable as observation service because there was no physician order for the service. This often affects payment for that stay since the comprehensive ambulatory payment classification (C-APC) payment for an observation stay requires eight or more hours of observation on the claim. It is for this reason that CC44 changes should be done as early as possible rather than waiting until near discharge. Conversely, one does not want to rush into the CC44 change too soon on some cases. For example, if a patient with chest pain was admitted as inpatient and is about to undergo their stress test, it would be wise to wait to see the results of that test before proceeding with the change. If the CC44 change is made to outpatient and then the stress test turns out abnormal and the patient stays hospitalized for another day, passing the second midnight, they have to once again be admitted as inpatient, creating added work and physician frustration.

If the attending physician disagrees with the determination and insists the patient remains an inpatient, a second physician member of the UR committee must review the case. If this second UR committee physician agrees with the attending, then the inpatient admission stands and is billed. This situation would be infrequent but is worth discussing at the full UR committee meeting as a learning experience for all. Remember, the determination is a complex medical decision, and rational physicians may disagree on the proper care. If the second UR committee physician determines that the admission was not medically necessary but the attending continues to refuse to make the change, the patient remains inpatient but the admission should be self-denied.

Self-denial and rebill

The self-denial process has been part of Medicare regulations for a long time. As outlined in 42 *CFR* 482.30, CMS expects the hospital to review the necessity of admissions and services. But the reality was that some things slip through the UR net and get billed despite the lack of medical necessity. Prior to 2013, if an admission was determined to be improper, the hospital could be required to submit a no-pay inpatient self-denial claim but could then bill for a limited number of services that were provided to the patient, such as diagnostic testing, implants, and dressings.

When CMS started the Recovery Audit Contractor (RAC) program, the RACs focused much of their attention on short-stay inpatient admissions, denying them and claiming that the services could have been provided as outpatient with observation services. When this occurred, hospitals had the full DRG payment recouped and were paid nothing for the care provided to the patient, even though the care was necessary but simply provided in what the RACs felt was the wrong status.

Then in a landmark court case, *O'Connor v CMS,* a federal judge ruled that O'Connor Hospital was entitled to payment for the care they provided as if it was furnished as outpatient. In response to this, CMS issued guidelines on self-denial and rebilling in two rules in 2013, CMS-1455-R and CMS-1599-F.

In these rules, and in subsequent transmittals, CMS laid out the self-denial process. They indicated first that the medical necessity of the admission must be determined by the formal UR process as specified under 42 *CFR* 482.30(d) or 42 *CFR* 485.641. This includes written notification to the physician, patient, and hospital within two days of the determination. The hospital would then process the claim as a Part A inpatient claim and submit that as a no-pay claim. This is the "self-denial" part of the process. Once that claim processes, the hospital would be able to "rebill" for the care, first by submitting an outpatient Part B claim for all services prior to the inpatient order and then an inpatient Part B claim for all services after the admission order. As can be seen, the self-denial and rebill process requires the preparation of three claims and delays final payment for potentially months rather than a single claim for an admission that was changed via the CC44 process that is paid in weeks.

Many hospitals have a process in place to review all Medicare short-stay inpatient admissions prior to claim submission to determine if a Part A claim is appropriate or if the admission should be reviewed for self-denial. These hospitals feel it is better to find these cases internally rather than waiting for a Medicare auditor to find the claim and deny it, perhaps leading to further audits and even extrapolation of their findings to a larger population of claims.

It should be noted that if a surgical inpatient admission is self-denied and rebilled, the hospital will be paid the same payment as if the surgery was done as outpatient from the outset. This is certainly preferable to submitting an inpatient claim and having it denied and then missing the timely filing deadline to get paid under Part B, resulting in no payment at all.

Note that in the vast majority of cases, a self-denied admission does not affect Part A payment for a SNF stay after the admission because the rebilling preserves the inpatient admission and merely shifts payment from Part A to Part B. The exception is an inpatient admission where it is determined that the sole purpose of the admission was to accrue a three-day inpatient stay to allow the patient access to the Part A SNF benefit. In egregious cases such as this, Part A payment for the SNF may be denied.

No issue generates more anger and confusion among Medicare beneficiaries than observation "status"—a hospital stay that is really not a hospital stay. But Medicare gives hospital executives little choice. The government and payers set the guidelines for admission and impose tough penalties if the auditors believe that the hospital wrongly admitted patients as inpatient. In addition, much of the confusion and frustration patients feel about observation dates back many years when observation stays often went for several days, patients owed 20% of the approved payments, and the days did not qualify for access to their Part A SNF benefit. Although the anger and confusion remain, the advent of the 2-midnight rule and the creation of a C-APC payment for observation not only eliminates the long observation stays but means the out-of-pocket costs to a patient for an observation stay are significantly less than the Part A deductible they incur on the first day of an inpatient stay. The other problem with this thinking is that the hospital does not admit patients—physicians do—and physicians are not currently penalized and hospital executives are loathe to hold them accountable. Nevertheless, in the case of a patient who has already been discharged, the determination that an inpatient admission was not medically necessary must be made. This is one of the reasons we strongly urge the collection and presentation of denial data to the UR committee. Physicians often have no idea that their patients' hospitalization costs were denied payment. Presenting them with the data may prompt careful thought the next time the ARS offers admission status advice.

Payment disparities

Continued-stay reviews also speak to the issue of physician and hospital payment. Back in 2012, 29% of licensed physicians worked in hospitals or in practices wholly or partially owned by hospitals. In 2019, that number increased to 47.4%. Buying practices and recruiting doctors out of residency is a popular strategy to ensure a consistent referral stream, and their value to the hospital has been borne out in several studies. Hospitalists are generally paid a salary with a risk sharing component, where if certain metrics, such as reduction in readmissions or costs per case, are achieved the physician will receive additional compensation. However, unless value-based contracts with payers are at play, claims for medical services provided by the hospitalists are still billed as traditional fee-for-service; that is, each visit to the patient's room generates a charge, even if the hospital is denied payment. As we mentioned earlier, back in 2014, CMS released *Medicare Program Integrity Transmittal 541*, which gave Medicare Administrative Contractors (MAC) and Zone Program Integrity Contractors (ZPIC) the discretion to deny payment to physicians if the hospital payment is denied. While it has not been invoked by MACs as of publication, it signals that CMS is willing to hold physicians financially responsible for their hospital admission and continued-stay decisions. Other, more recent regulation shows that CMS is taking tangible steps toward increasing physician financial accountability.

In July 2020, CMS started a mandatory prior authorization program for specific surgeries if performed in the outpatient hospital setting. They started with five cosmetic-like surgeries, such as blepharoplasty and panniculectomy, but added cervical spine fusion and implanted spinal neurostimulator in July 2021. In this program, prior authorization is a condition of payment, and CMS states that if it not obtained and the surgery proceeds, the hospital's claim and every physician claim will be denied. Unlike *Transmittal 541*, where the MAC and ZPIC have an option to deny associated claims, in this program it is required. These denials will include not only claims from the surgeon but also the pathologist, radiologist, and anesthesiologist. These doctors had no role in the process of obtaining the prior authorization or even determining the need for surgery. However, not only are they held responsible, but if their professional claim is denied, they must appeal it on their own and cannot "ride the coattails" of the hospital's appeal.

Stage 3: Duration of Stays: Continued-Stay Review

The *CoP* for UR require the hospital to review the medical necessity for admissions, the duration of stays, and the services provided, so the UR process does not end once a patient is hospitalized. While the *CoP* state that duration-of-stay reviews are reserved for cases that are "reasonably assumed to be outlier cases based on extended length of stay," the fact is that hospital UR staff review a lot of Medicare cases every day, whether they are suspected of being outliers or not.

Continued-stay reviews are performed to confirm that the patient continues to need inpatient hospital care. Such a decision can be made using the same collaborative standard as the initial decision to hospitalize.

Together with the UR specialist, the attending physician reviews the patient's current clinical condition and plans for future care to determine whether the patient must remain hospitalized to receive services and reduce risk, or to determine whether the patient can be safely treated in a lesser setting.

The decision to continue hospitalization or discharge the patient to a lower level of care is important not only for payment purposes but also for evaluating the quality of care provided and the patient's safety. Each additional day of hospital care subjects the patient to another day of potential risk. There is ample literature on the risk of medication errors and hospital-acquired infections, and the adverse effects of limited mobility that accompany hospitalization are also well known. Commercial criteria discharge screens provide an additional resource to help the UR specialist make recommendations to the physician about the need for continued stay based on best-practice readiness for discharge.

For many physicians, once a patient is hospitalized, it is easier to complete the evaluation and treatment of all of the patient's medical issues, as opposed to discharging the patient with the need for outpatient follow-up. This preference can be due to concerns that the patient will not follow through with needed testing, exposing the patient to medical risk and the physician to medical liability risk. These risks are compounded as more and more hospitalists are managing inpatient care, which has led to some loss of continuity in care. The hospitalist depends upon the primary care physician (PCP) to read the discharge summary thoroughly and to arrange needed follow-up testing. Similarly, the PCP depends on the hospitalist to indicate in the summary all follow-up tests that are needed, along with all tests that have been performed but for which results are not yet available.

Concerns about continued community care are not unfounded, and there is evidence that, absent any follow-up, avoidable ED visits and readmissions are inevitable. That risk may lessen as hospitals enter into risk-based contracts and care coordination across the continuum for the most vulnerable patients becomes part of provider expectations. In its 2019 White Paper on Hospital Case Management Practice, the Case Management Society of America promotes coordination across the continuum as a feature of contemporary case management programs, whether sponsored by the hospital or in collaboration with community-based providers (CMSA, 2019).

Continued-stay review for treatment of primary disease

Physicians use their clinical experience and training to determine whether a patient requires continued hospitalization for treatment of a condition that warranted admission or a condition that developed during admission. The UR specialist should use the criteria set, review the medical record, and discuss with the physician to determine whether continued stay in the hospital is warranted. If the justification of continued stay is not clearly delineated in the medical record, then the UR specialist should ask the physician to clarify the medical reason for continued stay so that other caregivers are aware of the physician's impression and plan and to note that the needed care cannot be safely provided in a lesser setting.

Seasoned UR specialists also know to speak to the patient's nurse or case manager to try to uncover other issues at play that may have influenced the physician's decision. Sometimes they find out that the patient asked the doctor not to discharge them because they have no way to get home till the weekend or prefer the warm environment of the hospital to the cold reality of a homeless shelter. Many times, social services may be a referral option, but at the least, a discussion with the hospitalist and the PA should ensue. Acute hospital care is the most expensive item in the healthcare industry and poses the most risk. As part of the strategy to lower costs, UR will remain an important component to encourage all providers to practice high-quality, efficient medicine and bring costs down to a socially acceptable levels.

Hospital stays are getting progressively shorter. Advances in medical technology, such as peripherally inserted central catheters with small programmable infusion pumps, allow patients to receive long courses of intravenous antibiotics on an ambulatory basis. Surgery patients are no longer receiving large doses of intravenous opioids, instead getting targeted nerve blocks to provide effective, localized pain relief. SNFs are increasingly willing to accept patients with complex medical needs, and new potent oral medications have contributed to shortened hospital stays.

For patients who are covered by Medicare, the patient's current status and the number of midnights that have already passed must be evaluated. Medicare allows continued inpatient hospitalization without medical necessity only when a patient requires Part A skilled nursing care at a SNF but there are no available SNF beds in the geographic region. This exception does not apply if there are no beds available at the patient's desired facility. The patient does not have the option of remaining in the hospital while waiting for bed availability at their choice of SNF if there are beds at other (albeit less desirable) facilities in the region. To expedite the patient choice process, a designated individual should identify the immediately available options using CMS' online star rating found through Medicare's Nursing Home Compare website and should share those options with the patient. In late 2019, CMS updated the discharge planning *CoP* to give the patient a more active role in their hospital and post-acute care. While the provisions of that rule are outside the duties of the UR specialist, these added requirements have the potential to increase patient uncertainty in choosing a provider and slowing down the transition to the next level of care.

Commercial insurers will look to national best practices when determining the need for continued hospitalization and approving additional days. Hospital executives should expect the same consideration from their medical staff. The idea that "we have always done it this way at this hospital" does not represent effective, patient-centered care and should not be tolerated. The decision to continue hospitalization should be based on the answer to the question, "What would the best hospital in the country do?" It also remains to be seen how the rapid growth of "hospital at home" programs during the COVID-19 pandemic will affect continued stays. As the ability to provide care to acutely ill patients outside of the walls of the hospital improves—demonstrated during the COVID-19 pandemic by the rise of hospital-at-home programs and sophisticated telehealth services—we may see payers who are unwilling to approve long in-hospital stays, putting added pressure on the UR staff and physicians to justify every day of every hospital stay.

Continued-stay review for additional testing

The need for additional testing on hospital patients generally falls into two categories:

1. Tests that are needed to follow up on an abnormal result (which led to hospitalization or which was found during the hospital stay)
2. Testing unrelated to the reason for hospitalization but is warranted

For the second category, differentiate whether the test must be done to assess the patient's stability for discharge, in which case the test is clearly indicated during the hospital stay. But if continued care in the hospital does not depend on the test results, the test could be deferred to the outpatient setting. An often-cited study of trauma patients who underwent whole-body CT scans found over 40% had incidental findings, often called "incidentalomas," and over half of them were not clinically significant (Fakler, Ozkurtul, and

Josten, 2014). Thyroid and pulmonary nodules are commonly found on CT scans of the chest, and hepatic and adrenal lesions are the most prevalent finding in CT scans of the abdomen. These incidental lesions rarely require evaluation during the hospitalization. Beyond radiographic abnormalities, many patients who are ill will also have incidental laboratory abnormalities.

The physician should evaluate the need for follow-up testing while the patient remains hospitalized within the clinical and psychosocial context of the hospitalization. In most cases, the testing can and should be deferred to the outpatient setting. However, if for example a potentially malignant mass was found incidentally in a patient who is homeless and is therefore unlikely to follow up, further testing during the hospital stay may be warranted, with compelling medical documentation to support the physician's decision.

If a patient needs testing unrelated to the hospitalization, there is no medical reason to have the test performed while he or she is hospitalized even though doing so might be more convenient for the patient. This testing, called "while you are here" testing, is often used to complete tests such as an overdue mammogram. However, the patient's inpatient care should be solely directed to the illness that warranted hospitalization. There is no additional reimbursement to the hospital for most "while you are here" testing, and remaining in the hospital for such tests just adds to the clinical risk inherent in any hospital stay.

■ **Figure 6.1**

Case study for continuing-stay utilization review

A 67-year-old female was hospitalized as an inpatient with a severe exacerbation of her emphysema. She was treated with nebulized medications and intravenous steroids. Her admitting laboratories included a hemoglobin of 11.8 mg/dL (normal 12.0–14.5). On hospital day four, her breathing was better, and she was stable for discharge from the pulmonary point of view, but her hemoglobin was now 11.6 mg/dL. She had no signs of bleeding.

Her physician consulted a gastroenterologist for anemia. The gastroenterologist scheduled the patient for a colonoscopy the next day and ordered a polyethylene glycol-electrolyte preparation, which consists of the patient drinking 2 liters of fluid in the evening and 2 liters in the morning. That evening, the patient had difficulty drinking the fluid and had several episodes of emesis. The next morning, she was only able to drink less than 1 liter of the fluid, and the gastroenterologist rescheduled the colonoscopy for the next day, placing the patient on a clear liquid diet and ordering a repeat of the prep. The next day, the gastroenterologist completed the colonoscopy, which was normal. In the recovery room, the patient was slow to awaken after sedation and her blood pressure was low, so she was kept an additional day to recover.

In this case, the patient had mild anemia, and a colonoscopy was indicated to evaluate for a colonic lesion, but there was no indication to perform it during her hospitalization. As noted, she had difficulty with the preparation, and the procedure was delayed one day. She also had complications post-procedure, extending her stay an additional day. If the UR specialist had been notified that the physician had consulted gastroenterology for a nonurgent colonoscopy, he or she could have worked with the doctors and patient to schedule the test to take place after discharge. Performing the colonoscopy during the patient's hospital stay not only resulted in complications but also extended her hospital stay by two days. There was no additional reimbursement to the hospital for the procedure or other services provided to the patient during those days, including room charges and nursing services.

Continued-stay and level of care

A patient may be cared for in various locations throughout a hospital stay. Critically ill patients or those requiring advanced technologies are cared for in the intensive care units. Patients requiring cardiac rhythm monitoring and less critically ill patients are often cared for on telemetry units, and patients receiving routine hospital care are cared for on the medical and surgical units. The physician usually decides on which service unit the patient will receive care, based partially on objective patient needs but often influenced by subjective factors, such as the physician's comfort with the nursing care in that area, the care received by their patients in the past, the nursing staffing ratios, and, occasionally, by adverse past experience.

As can be expected, the cost of a day in the intensive care unit is much higher than the cost of a day on a telemetry unit, which in turn is more expensive than a day on a general medical-surgical unit. As a result, physicians should place patients in the area that can best meet—but not exceed—their needs. Many hospitals have developed criteria for the use of critical care and telemetry units and have given the medical director of those units the authority to order transfer of patients out of the unit to a more appropriate lower level of care. Another method is to require the physician to reorder the use of telemetry on a daily basis so that there is a conscious decision made that it is needed. Closed critical care and step-down units managed by intensivists have grown in popularity as a political strategy to prevent misuse by the medical staff. It can also be argued that patients under the care of an intensivist in the intensive care unit (ICU) will receive better, more evidence-based care.

Accountable care units (ACU) dedicated exclusively to specific patient populations have appeared in several facilities to overcome these political hotspots. For example, many hospitals have created "one stop" ACUs for the cardiac patient who is attended to by the same care team from admission to transition, thus avoiding intra-hospital transfers and setting the stage for team-based, value-added incentive programs based on patient care and performance outcomes. These specialized units typically have lower patient-to-nurse ratios to meet the increased needs of the patient without requiring an intensive care unit. This strategy is also being used in large academic medical centers for major transplant cases where treatment plans have been standardized by the medical staff. The advantage of these ACUs, like their ambulatory care accountable care organization cousins, is having an accountable team responsible for managing care, services, and resources throughout the patient's hospitalization.

Continued-stay review and the PA

The PA role in continued-stay reviews is similar to admission reviews.

The UR specialist reviews medical documentation to support the patient's need for continued hospitalization as well as level of care (does the patient still need to be in ICU or telemetry?). Using documentation in concert with criteria guidelines, a determination is made about the patient's need for continued hospital care. If documentation does not support continued stay and a conversation with the attending physician does not result in information that supports medical necessity for continued stay, a secondary review by the PA is warranted.

Many EHR systems have the capacity to include clinical guidelines in the form of decision-support tools. This technology accelerates the search for key clinical data and should change the future focus of UR. However, we anticipate that the addition of artificial intelligence (AI) solutions will further enhance the process through the use of learning algorithms, which will reduce the need for concurrent reviews. The promise of AI is great, but like many new services, promise does not always translate into actual beneficial clinical results. As the number of products and uses increase, it will be important to ensure these products work as advertised and use a database that truly represents the patient population on which the product is being used. For example, an AI program developed to screen for melanoma was based on a patient population that was predominantly white, ignoring the incidence of melanoma in people of color (Noor, 2020).

To date, many physicians view UR as an effort to limit their professional autonomy, and possibly their income, and it is not uncommon to hear reports that hospitalists go out of their way to avoid contact with the UR team. Clearly, UR must evolve from its current role as a "command and control" regulatory program to more of an educational and decision support system for physicians. In this way, UR will be of greater value to practitioners and patients and, as a result, should gain broader support. As we have mentioned before, it must start with a better onboarding program for every medical student, intern, and resident so that they have a better understanding of the oversight agencies and payers that continue to influence their practice decisions.

Continued-stay review and throughput

For many years, the UR team and case managers were asked to capture data on progression of care delays (PoCD) and potentially avoidable days (PAD), referred to as "throughput" in today's vernacular, which account for a large portion of extended length of stay. Those reports often sat in dusty binders or electronic folders in the UR office. But once UR leaders learned how to present the data in financial terms, they were further refined for greater specificity and became essential to identify throughput bottlenecks and who was causing them. They are now part of every UR committee's review of progression of care issues.

Just as the actions of physicians contribute to inefficiency, so, too, does the work of hospital associates in every department. Inefficiencies abound, whether it is from a delay by the transporter moving a patient from ICU to telemetry or the delay caused by incorrect face sheet (demographics) information. According to management expert Peter Drucker, hospitals are the most chaotic and complex of organizations. The hospital environment houses a confluence of multiple professions that must work together to provide economically responsible activities in the service of the patient. Compounding this complexity is the realization that most of the hospital's professionals have not been taught how to work within a cooperative framework; each profession tends to view itself both as unique and competing for resources without surrendering control over its respective fiefdoms.

Although efficiency is essential for success, ingrained organizational factors often cause progression-of-care failure. A real-life example involves hospital A, which, in an effort to market its expanded imaging service product line, prioritized outpatient requests for imaging studies during weekday daytime hours. However, this new initiative was a hardship for working patients who couldn't take time off from work. Additionally, no one considered the downstream effects of the change, the most significant being a deliberate delay in scheduling inpatients till after 4 p.m., which resulted in an uptick in length of stay. The hospital's marketing department is supposed to organize responsiveness to the community needs, and in this case, information from the community about scheduling needs would have been beneficial to the hospital. Instead, inadequate communication with the consumers and the lack of involvement of stakeholders in the planning process led to implementation of an unsuccessful initiative.

This is not an isolated example of hospital inefficiency and why staff often describe hospitals as operationally dysfunctional organizations. We are sure that our readers can contribute many more examples from their hospitals about decisions that are being made without considering the implications beginning, as explained earlier, with the individual negotiating contracts without giving any thought to the UR language and its downstream consequences. Isaac Newton's axiom that every action has an equal and opposite reaction should be part of the planning and analysis for every new initiative.

Efficient progression of care is a product of the processes in place: "Processes are the chains of linked activities that take inputs and transform them into value-added outputs" (Beckham, 1996). In the example about hospital A, the new processes undermined the desired outcomes and sacrificed value. According to W. Edwards Deming, the pioneering expert on performance improvement, more than 85% of organizational problems are process related, whereas only 15% or less can be blamed on the people who carry out the process activities (Walton, 1986). Process improvement is still on every hospital executive's mind, but despite recent incarnations of Deming's Plan, Do, Study, Act improvement cycle, such as Lean, Six Sigma, or Kaizen projects, hospital inefficiencies still exist. UR specialists, with their frontline experience, are well positioned to contribute their insights and information to process improvement activities.

Progression of care, or throughput, has been an ongoing battle for decades. Attendance at a recent hospital process improvement committee highlights the ongoing problems with progression of care when one of the committee members reported that "seems like we've been meeting for 30 years and nothing has changed." He may have been exaggerating, but every hospital associate knows that outstanding patient care outcomes result from the processes created to deliver patient care. However, those processes are fraught with obstacles. In many organizations, nurses and case managers spend a large portion of their time trying to overcome the obstacles that UR specialists identify as impeding the throughput and delaying discharge. Although performance improvement initiatives generally originate in the quality management or performance improvement departments, case managers, nurses, and UR specialists can easily identify and quantify system snags that warrant the attention of leadership and of the responsible department head by capturing and quantifying progression of care delays and potentially avoidable days.

The fundamental purpose of capturing PoCDs and PADs is to identify ways to improve throughput and to hold delivery-of-care process owners accountable for outcomes. Many executives automatically point fingers at discharge processes as the primary cause of throughput delays. But once this PAD process is in place, that assumption can be disputed.

Although PoCDs and PADs are a cost issue in the C-suite, they are primarily a quality issue for the patient. This distinction is important. The ability of the nurse, case manager, or UR specialist to effectively reduce these impediments and move the patient through the acute episode of care will be undermined if the physician believes they are only lobbying to expedite the patient's care in an effort to save money for the hospital. The incentive for the physician to engage in efforts to improve throughput must be an interest in maintaining the patient's quality of care, avoiding patient risk (either financial or clinical), or some personal vested interest.

A structured approach to capture, quantify, and disseminate trends in progression-of-care performance is a relatively simple process, but it is best to sketch out this approach on paper before creating it in an electronic format. Begin the process by identifying all the possible reasons that a PoCD or PAD might occur. It's not unusual to compile a list of more than 150 items, including delays caused by an incomplete or inaccurate face sheet, inability to get a timely stress test or MRI on a weekend, unavailability of a radiologist to read an imaging study, or an avoidable day because the admitting physician refused to discharge without the consent of the consulting physician.

Be specific about the delay. For example, an item listed as a "delay in test results" does not give the source of the delay and is therefore not actionable. However, noting a "delay in radiology test results" provides actionable information, as the specificity of this information allows the team to know where to start when attempting to solve the problem (in this case, have a discussion with the radiology department manager). Once all items are identified, categorize them into four areas based on the following issues:

- Those that can be attributed to patients
- Those that can be attributed to physicians
- Those that can be attributed to ancillary providers
- Those that are system-related

Figure 6.2 is a sample report listing 40 system-related issues that a UR team identified as causing PoCDs and/or PADs and that may ultimately delay timely discharge.

■ **Figure 6.2**

	Sample progression-of-care delays and potentially avoidable days capture form					
S codes	**System occurrences**		**Date of occurrence**	**Was action taken to avoid progression-of-care delays or potentially avoidable days?**		**Comments**
				Yes	No	
	Incomplete/inaccurate registration demographics					
	Delay in phlebotomy service					
	Laboratory test results report delay					
	Electromyogram not available on weekend					
	Critical care bed not available					
	Telemetry bed not available					
	Medical/surgical bed not available					
	Intravenous equipment not available					
	Therapy not available on weekend					
	Surgery not done on weekend					
	Delay in receiving approval (authorization) to transfer patient to another facility/lower level of care					
	Facility refuses transfer over weekend/holiday					
	Skilled nursing facility (SNF) bed not available					
	Rehabilitation bed not available					
	Awaiting paperwork (Medicaid application, pre-admission screening, and resident review)					
	Transportation not available					
	Meal delivered to NPO patient					
	Integrated delivery system partner unwilling to accept patient					

S codes	System occurrences	Date of occurrence	Was action taken to avoid progression-of-care delays or potentially avoidable days?		Comments
			Yes	No	
	Unable to find community resource for follow-up visit				
	Delay in transferring to hospital-based rehab/SNF unit				
	Commercial payer refuses to deliver notice of noncoverage				
	Delay in CT scan/MRI schedule				
	Delay in cystoscopy schedule				
	Delay in angiography schedule				
	Delay in percutaneous endoscopic gastrostomy placement by medical doctor				
	Delay in discharge readiness evaluation due to physical therapy				
	Delay in ordering physical medicine and rehabilitation consult				
	Delay in availability to insert peripherally inserted central catheter line				
	Delay in physical/occupational therapy initial evaluation				
	Delay in swallowing evaluation				
	Unavailable service or delay in treatment to psychiatric drug/alcohol unit/facility				
	Delay in physician advisor response to medical necessity issue				
	Delay in physician advisor response to quality/safety issue				
	No exercise stress test on weekends				
	Imaging test not available after 4 p.m. or weekend				
	Awaiting guardianship				
	Delay in durable medical equipment delivery				
	Delay in financial counselor response				
	Nursing delay to refer discharge plan to post-acute transition center for processing				

Source: Phoenix Medical Management, Inc., in Pompano Beach, Florida. Reprinted with permission.

Financially quantify PoCDs and PADs

Once all the possible reasons for a delay in throughput are identified, ask the CFO to identify a metric that can be used to quantify the financial implication of PoCDs and PADs. The most commonly used metrics are the average charge or cost per patient day or the average revenue per patient day. It really doesn't matter so long as the metric is used consistently. To pilot the new system, ask each member of the case management, UR, and clinical documentation integrity (CDI) teams to track these delays for each patient, either manually via a paper form or with the system built into many case management systems. Have them check off when they believe a PoCD or PAD may have occurred and whether they did anything to overcome the problem. Any day or portion of a day that in some way can be perceived by the patient, the payer, or the physician as unnecessary or noncontributory qualifies as a delay and potentially avoidable day and subjects the patient to avoidable risk. The most expensive resource commonly provided by the hospital is an avoidable day, and the costs associated with it will never be recovered.

Remember that each member of this trio will encounter PoCDs and PADs from a different perspective. Case managers will encounter PoCDs as they round with the physicians and clinical team or if they are trying to expedite a discharge, whereas the UR specialists and the CDI team are more likely to encounter PoCDs or a PAD as a result of their medical record review or access management activities.

At regular intervals, generate a report containing all or some of the fields. If data is captured routinely and consistently, trends and patterns will appear within three to four months, and items with minimal occurrences can be removed, allowing for a reduction in the volume of items. A monthly occurrence does not generally constitute a trend. Once the list is narrowed down to the top 25–30 items and access to an electronic counterpart is available in the EHR, the UR manager should collaborate with the information techs at the hospital to determine how to best make the capture process as simple as possible. It is worth repeating that it is key to not only track the delay but to attribute it to the correct party. If the payer takes 72 hours to approve transfer to a SNF, that delay cannot be attributed to the physician since they had no role in signing the contract that allowed the payer to take those 72 hours. But if a patient's discharge is delayed a day because the physician does not round until 9 p.m., that would be attributed to the physician.

Figure 6.3 is a sample of a useful PoCD/PAD report generated from data downloaded from Access® into an Excel® spreadsheet. Not only does it provide the source and volume of delays and avoidable days, but it quantifies them financially. Note the report's inclusion of dollars saved/recovered as a result of an action taken by a member of the case management or UR team. This piece of information is essential in the development process. If the individual identifying the PoCD or PADs subsequently took action to avoid or overcome the obstacle, there must be a mechanism in place to quantify that action, as it has a direct bearing on the value that the individual brings to the desired outcome and the program.

▪ Figure 6.3

					Sample progression-of-care delays and potentially avoidable days report			
	Code	**Description**	**Source**	**PAD**	**Potentially lost revenue**	**Avoided**	**Recovered/ Saved**	**Net outcome**
June	N1,N2,N3	Rx not transcribed	Nursing	67	282,941	22	92,906	190,035
June	S9	No W/E Surgery	OR	41	173,143	0	0	173,143
June	S5	Step-down bed n/a	System	32	135,136	7	29,561	105,575
June	S12	Med nec not docu	Med staff	31	130,913	17	71,791	59,122
June	D11	Preop day	Med staff	24	101,352	2	8,446	92,906
June	CC3	Counselor not avail	System	17	71,791	2	8,446	63,345
June	D8	On call MD won't DC	Med staff	17	71,791	11	46,453	25,338
June	D9	Inadeq docu for inpt LOC	Med staff	12	50,676	8	33,784	16,892
June	D4	Test unrelated to adm	Med staff	14	59,122	6	25,338	33,784
June	N5	Incorrect face sheet	System	32	135,136	7	29,561	105,575
				June totals:	1,212,001		346,286	865,715
July	N1,N2,N3	Rx not transcribed	Nursing	54	228,042	17	71,791	156,251
July	S9	No W/E Surgery	OR	50	211,150	0	0	211,150
July	D11	Preop day	Med staff	24	101,352	1	4,223	97,129
July	S5	Step down bed n/a	System	19	80,237	3	12,669	67,568
July	S12	Med nec not docu	Med staff	22	92,906	19	80,237	12,669
July	D9	Inade docu for LOC	Med staff	18	76,014	10	42,230	33,784
July	D8	On call MD won't DC	Med staff	16	67,568	11	46,453	21,115
July	CC3	Counselor not avail	System	11	46,453	0	0	46,453
July	D5	Consult delay	Med staff	7	29,561	1	4,223	25,338
July	P3	Patient ref avail SNF	Patient	6	25,338	0	0	25,338
				July totals:	958,621		261,826	696,795
	Code	**Description**	**Source**	**PAD**	**Potentially lost revenue**	**Avoided**	**Recovered/ Saved**	**Net outcome**
Aug	N1,N2,N3	Rx not transcribed	Nursing	47	198,481	21	88,683	109,798
Aug	S9	No W/E surgery	OR	44	185,812	0	0	185,812
Aug	S12	Med nec not docu	Med staff	27	114,021	17	71,791	42,230
Aug	D11	Preop day	Med staff	27	114,021	2	8,446	105,575
Aug	S5	Step-down bed n/a	System	18	76,014	2	8,446	67,568
Aug	D9	Inade docu for LOC	Med staff	12	50,676	11	46,453	4,223
Aug	A7	Delayed lab rep	Lab	7	29,561	5	21,115	8,446
Aug	CC3	Counselor not avail	System	6	25,338	3	12,669	12,669
Aug	D8	On call MD won't DC	Med staff	7	29,561	4	16,892	12,669
Aug	A8	Delayed rad report	Radiology	6	25,338	4	16,892	8,446
				August totals:	848,823		291,387	557,436
				YTD	$3,019,445		$899,499	$2,119,946

Source: Phoenix Medical Management, Inc., in Pompano Beach, Florida. Reprinted with permission.

Consider the following guidelines when developing a method of measuring progression-of-care efficiency:

- Data must be consistently captured, quantified, and disseminated.
- Capture both delays and days using a predetermined standard of measurement. Generally, any event that results or may result in a delay of four hours or less should be recorded as half day.
- As trends begin to emerge, narrow the list of items to those that are high-risk, high-volume, or high-cost issues.
- Remind team members that PoCDs and PADs do not have to be justified. For example, no further explanation is needed if a delay is anticipated because a physician orders a test unrelated to the reason for the patient's inpatient admission; just record it and attribute it.
- Disseminate the report monthly to everyone involved, including the process owner, medical staff, executive team, and UR committee.
- Post graphic visuals of the outcomes to demonstrate efficiency improvement over time and the effect of case management and UR program initiatives.

If everyone connected with the patient's progression-of-care activities participates in this process, capturing saved days can be used to demonstrate a program's return on investment. In the sample report, the team avoided potential costs of more than $250,000 per month, so this process can provide a significant financial benefit for the facility. It is also important to provide feedback to the team. If the data determined that lack of MRIs on weekends resulted in a significant number of avoidable days and administration decided to approve bringing in a technologist on weekends, the team should be told that their diligence in collecting data resulted in a process change.

Continued-stay review and outlier certification

As part of the 2015 Outpatient Prospective Payment System final rule, CMS modified paragraph (a) of 42 *CFR* §424.13 to require inpatient continued-stay certification for patients who remain in the hospital more than 20 days. Prior to the 20th day of the hospitalization, the UR specialist must remind the physician that documentation in the medical record needs to justify why that patient continues to require care in the hospital as opposed to a lesser setting, such as a SNF or at home. Specifically, the physicians must document:

1. The reasons for either: a) Continued hospitalization of the patient for medical treatment or medically required diagnostic study; or b) special or unusual services for cost outlier cases such as participation in clinical trials or testing of new technologies. If the patient still requires care that could be provided in a sub-acute facility, such as a SNF, but there is no accepting facility in the area, the continuing stay can be certified but the physician note should indicate that a search for an accepting SNF is ongoing. There is no specific form or statement required and the information can be inferred from the physician's written discussion of the patient's conditions and treatment plans. For example, "septic shock with hypotension, continue pressors" meets the requirement, as patients in septic shock require hospital care. On the other hand, if documentation states that the patient is "alert and oriented, in no distress, ambulating in hallways," there is no intrinsic reason for continued hospital care, so the notes must clearly support the continued stay.

2. The second required element is the estimated time that the patient will need to spend in the hospital. Although this may be part of the physician progress notes, the physician should be asked to document an estimated LOS. This estimation does not need to be accurate; the physician can make an educated guess in days or weeks and document that. For example, the physician could

document that he or she expects the patient to stay two more weeks. If the estimate is wrong, then there are no consequences, as CMS does not expect physicians to have a crystal ball.

3. The plans for post-hospital care, if appropriate. This documentation should be regularly recorded but must be in the record as day 20 approaches to ensure that the conditions and treatment that require hospital care are clearly described. Note that the regulation states "no later than" day 20, which means that certification can be performed on any day prior to day 20 if it is anticipated that the patient will remain hospitalized on day 20. We suggest setting up a tickler file in your UR software application to remind the UR specialist, CDI team member, or case manager to speak with the attending physician about this requirement.

Critical access hospitals also have a certification requirement. CMS expects physicians to certify that the patient may reasonably expect to be discharged or transferred within 96 hours of admission. CMS goes on to say that all physician certification requirements must occur no later than one day before the date on which the claim for inpatient service is submitted. This is unrelated to the outlier payment threshold but rather is related to the requirement that critical access hospitals only admit patients who have an expected inpatient stay of under 96 hours.

Medicare pays hospitals outlier payments to protect facilities from excessive losses stemming from cases in which care costs are abnormally high for Medicare beneficiaries. The program determines if a hospital qualifies for an inpatient outlier payment using a complex formula using a cost-to-charge ratio threshold; for fiscal year 2021, the inpatient outlier payment is $29,064. The actual payment to the hospital is 80% of the incurred costs that exceed the threshold, so while there is an additional payment, that amount does not cover the complete cost of care. There is also an outlier payment system that likewise provides an added payment above a specified threshold, but in this situation, the hospital receives only 50% of the costs that exceed the threshold.

Stage 4: Post-Acute Activities—Denials and Appeals

Never has there been a more critical time for revenue cycle leaders to identify ways to increase cash flow and stop revenue leakage. The COVID-19 pandemic exacerbated current challenges, such as rising healthcare prices and nursing staff labor, and brought new obstacles to the forefront. Prior to the pandemic, 21% of hospitals reported $10 million or more in bad debt, but the AHA estimates that hospitals incurred more than $202 billion in losses due to a combination of reduced revenue and increased costs during the pandemic (AHA, 2020).

An effective revenue cycle not only requires an understanding of how to negotiate payer contracts but depends on familiarity with the complex and proprietary rules of each federal, state, and private insurance company, knowledge of correct coding and timely filing methodologies, experience appealing rejected or denied claims, and application of best practices for tracking and monitoring cases. Monitoring claims, using past experiences with denied claims, often means putting holds on claims containing selected, denial-risky principal diagnoses before sending out the claim—chest pain being the classic example. Every appeal team coordinator knows that a principal diagnosis of chest pain will almost automatically trigger a denial for an inpatient claim. Generally, this occurs when the Health Level 7 interface messaging system, which is used to prepare the hospital claim form UB-04, is pulling the information for the claim form from the initial presenting diagnosis or chief complaint field on the registration form rather than the final diagnosis field in the

EHR. It should be noted that there are rare occasions where chest pain can be the principal diagnosis for an inpatient admission, but these should all be reviewed presubmission.

Denial prevention

Denial management is, in our opinion, an oxymoron. Have you ever heard of a fall management program or a medication error management program? No, of course not. Organizational efforts always focus on how to prevent falls and medication errors; the same should hold true for denials. They must be prevented to avoid all the backroom fixes, rework, and revenue delays that otherwise accumulate. To prevent denials—just like falls and medication errors—a root-cause analysis via the EDI 835 remittances of where, when, and why the denials occurred must be performed to expose trends, uncover hidden problems, and create work lists to route denied claims to the appropriate biller's desk.

A denial prevention culture begins with understanding the scope of the problem, which requires an accurate denial rate. To compute your hospital's denial rate, start with A) the total claims filed to a specific payer—both the number of claims and charge amounts. Then B) calculate the number and total dollar charges of denied claims. Finally, calculate your denial percentage by dividing B by A. We recommend two calculations: one based on first-pass denial information and the second based on final disposition of a claim after all appeals have been exhausted.

A denial is any situation where a payment for a claim is less than the amount that was contractually agreed for the services rendered. There are soft denials that have the potential to be paid if the provider takes timely follow-up action. In these cases, an appeal is not required but timely action is. Examples include pending receipt of medical records, missing or inaccurate claims information, or coding or charge errors.

Hard denials are those that result in revenue that is lost or written off. There are two kinds of hard denials: those that were avoidable and resulted from inaction on the part of the hospital and those where the insurer's final decision not to pay a claim resulted from lack of preauthorization, the services were not covered by the patient's insurance contract, or the claim was filed too late. Hard denials must be appealed.

According to the Change Healthcare 2020 Revenue Cycle Denials Index, 11.1% of claims were denied upon initial submission and "[h]alf of all denials are caused by front-end revenue cycle issues with registration and eligibility approaching 27% of denials." Other front-end denials include authorization and services that were not covered by the patient's benefit package. In total, according to the report, about half of denials—49.7%—are caused by front-end revenue cycle issues.

Clinical denials are those that result from the absence of medical necessity, incorrect status, or noncovered services determined by National Coverage Determination, Local Coverage Determination, or payer policy. Medicare denials have gone through the payer's adjudication system and have been reviewed and denied for clinical cause. Depending on the language of the commercial contract, payers may issue a complete denial, carve out a day or service, or change the admission to observation (which a commercial payer might say is not really a denial—just a lower payment). They might downgrade an intensive care unit day to an acute day and an acute admission to a skilled nursing day. In 2020, hospitals reported an exponential increase in the automatic downgrading of both facility and professional charges for emergency department visits. In fact, one payer proposed in June 2021 to deny all claims for ED visits where their proprietary algorithm determines that the patient did not have a true emergency. This proposal was delayed when the uproar from the medical community spread to the national media (AHA, 2021).

These coding downgrades are often difficult to detect. For example, the hospital will submit a claim for a level 4 ED visit, and the payer will run their algorithm and determine the "correct" level is 3 and simply issue a payment for a level 3 visit. When this payment is received by the patient finance office, the difference between the billed level 4 amount and the paid level 3 payment may simply be posted as a "contractual adjustment" without anyone realizing they did not get the expected level 4 contracted payment and it should have been correctly posted as a denial. This tactic, whether intentional or not, is not unusual, and it is only by working with revenue cycle leaders that the source of the shift from "denial" to "contractual adjustment" is uncovered. With all of this considered, it cannot be overstressed that contract language matters!

Electronic remittances: The source of truth

Objective information produced by electronic data is fast becoming an essential component of value-based care and permeates every component of the healthcare ecosystem. Although silos and roadblocks may prevent effective data sharing, there are outputs that would add value to the work of the UR specialist and that should be accessible to every hospital leader. The most valuable of these—and often the most elusive—are reports on payer denials.

In enacting HIPAA, Congress mandated the establishment of federal standards for the security of protected health information (PHI). The purpose of HIPAA is to ensure that every covered entity has implemented safeguards to protect the confidentiality, integrity, and availability of electronic PHI, and HIPAA gives patients an array of rights with respect to that information. At the same time, HIPAA expressly permits disclosure of PHI needed for patient care, treatment, payment, or healthcare operations.

The original intent of HIPAA was administrative simplification. HIPAA required the Secretary of HHS to adopt standards to support the electronic exchange of administrative and financial healthcare transactions. These transactions primarily occur between healthcare providers and health insurance plans or clearinghouses. The standards, specified by HIPAA 5010 requirements for the electronic transmission of healthcare payment and benefit information, enabled health information to be exchanged computer-to-computer through an electronic data interchange (EDI).

The enigma of the 837 and 835

There's an old maxim in both business and medicine that says "you can't manage what you don't measure." This is especially true of payer denial information. Without gathering and analyzing all the necessary data and knowing the source of the leakage, the organization is hamstrung when it comes to preventing future denials. Actual denial information provides essential insights into the source of the denial and puts the onus on an accountable process owner to remedy the issues cited. Without denial information, there is very little that the UR specialist can do to prevent the denials in the first place. In the world of payer denial data, this means accessing and analyzing the valuable information contained in first pass EDI 835 payer remittances.

Two of the electronic data submission standards that were adopted with the passing of HIPAA are of particular interest to those involved in UR activities. The first is the EDI Health Care Claim Transaction set (EDI 837), which is used to submit the hospital's claim billing information either directly or via intermediary billers and claims clearinghouses. It can also be used to transmit healthcare claims and billing payment information between payers with different payment responsibilities where coordination of benefits is required. It is the standard submission of a hospital claim form.

The second electronic data submission standard, the EDI Health Care Claim Payment/Advice Transaction Set (EDI 835), is used by the payer to make a payment, send an Explanation of Benefits (EOB), send an Explanation of Payments (EOP) remittance advice, or make a payment and send an EOP remittance advice from a health insurer to a healthcare provider either directly or via a financial institution.

These transaction sets are quite complex and using them as a source file for analytic purposes poses numerous reporting challenges. The 835 wasn't built with analytics and reporting in mind, which is why many organizations either don't use them, outsource with third-party analytic firms, or purchase EDI translator software.

The EDI 835 details the payment for each claim. A particular EDI 835 document may not necessarily match up one-for-one with a specific EDI 837. In fact, it is not uncommon for multiple EDI 835 transactions to be used in response to a single EDI 837 or for one EDI 835 to address multiple EDI 837 submissions. As a result, the EDI 835 is important to the patient financial services (PFS) office to track information about payments received for services provided and billed by the hospital, including the following:

- What charges were paid, reduced, or denied
- Whether there was a deductible, coinsurance, copay, etc.
- Any bundling or splitting of claims or line items
- How the payment was made, such as through a clearinghouse

There are three primary sets of codes used on the EOB. Claims Adjustment Group Codes (CAGC) consist of two alpha characters that identify general categories of denials. There are five EOB CAGCs: CO = contractual obligation, CR = corrections and reversals, OA = other adjustments, PI = payer-initiated reductions, and PR = patient responsibility.

The Claim Adjustment Reason Codes (CARC) and Remittance Advice Remark Codes (RARC) are part of the data contained in the EDI 835. The CARC conveys information about remittance processing, meaning that the payer must communicate why a claim was paid differently than it was billed. If there is no adjustment to a claim/line, then there is no adjustment reason code. The RARCs are used to provide additional information to explain the CARC.

CMS maintains the CARC and RARC lists, which are updated three times a year (in early March, July, and November), are developed by X12, an American National Standards Institute organization, and are published by Washington Publishing Company. There are hundreds of codes explaining why a claim was denied—whether for technical errors, benefit limitations, or clinical issues. Here are a few examples of the CARCs (*https://x12.org/codes/claim-adjustment-reason-codes*):

- 4—The procedure code is inconsistent with the modifier used.
- 10—The diagnosis is inconsistent with the patient's gender.
- 24—Charges are covered under a capitation agreement/managed care plan.
- 60—Charges for outpatient services are not covered when performed within a period of time prior to or after inpatient services.
- 95—Plan procedures not followed.
- 117—Transportation is only covered to the closest facility that can provide the necessary care.
- 150—Payer deems the information submitted does not support this level of service.
- 163—Attachment/other documentation referenced on the claim was not received.
- 167—This diagnosis is not covered.

- 186—Level of care change adjustment.
- 197—Precertification/authorization/notification/pretreatment absent.
- 210—Payment adjusted because pre-certification not received in a timely fashion.
- 226—Information requested from the billing/rendering provider was not provided or not provided timely or was insufficient/incomplete.
- 242—Services not provided by network/primary care providers.
- 249—This claim has been identified as a readmission.

And here are a few examples of RARC codes (*https://x12.org/codes/remittance-advice-remark-codes*):

- M42—The medical necessity form must be personally signed by the attending physician.
- M60—Missing certificate of medical necessity.
- MA36—Missing/incomplete/invalid patient name.
- MA43—Missing/incomplete/invalid patient status.
- MA66—Missing/incomplete/invalid principal procedure code.
- MA96—Claim rejected. Coded as a Medicare Managed Care Demonstration, but patient is not enrolled in a Medicare managed care plan.
- N115—This decision was based on a Local Coverage Determination (LCD). An LCD provides a guide to assist in determining whether a particular item or service is covered.
- N143—The patient was not in a hospice program during all or part of the service dates billed.
- N208—Missing/incomplete/invalid DRG code.
- N227—Incomplete/invalid certificate of medical necessity.

In accordance with HIPAA 5010 ERA standards, coded data from the insurer to the provider is transmitted via an XML report. The complexity of the XML is compounded because so many commercial insurers and states use their own format and versions of the codes.

Figure 6.4 is an actual sample of an 835 ERA from one payer. As you can see, because the report is transmitted in XML format, practical use of the data is daunting.

■ Figure 6.4

Sample of an 835 ERA

```xml
<?xml version="1.0" encoding="UTF-8"?>
<ediroot>
    <interchange Standard="ANSI X.12" Date="160125" Time="2359"
        Version="00501" Control="602500086">
        <sender>
            <address Id="12102           " Qual="ZZ" />
        </sender>
        <receiver>
            <address Id="1926706         " Qual="29" />
        </receiver>
        <group GroupType="HP" ApplSender="12102" ApplReceiver="1926706'
            Date="20160125" Time="2359" Control="86" StandardCode="X"
            StandardVersion="005010X221A1">
            <transaction DocType="835" Name="Health Care Claim Payment/
                Control="000000003">
                <segment Id="BPR">
                    <element Id="BPR01">I</element>
                    <element Id="BPR02">23454.29</element>
                    <element Id="BPR03">C</element>
                    <element Id="BPR04">ACH</element>
                    <element Id="BPR05">CCP</element>
                    <element Id="BPR06">01</element>
                    <element Id="BPR07">081517693</element>
                    <element Id="BPR08">DA</element>
                    <element Id="BPR09">152302017081</element>
                    <element Id="BPR10">1205296137</element>
                    <element Id="BPR12">01</element>
                    <element Id="BPR13">031100092</element>
                    <element Id="BPR14">DA</element>
                    <element Id="BPR15">26728770</element>
                    <element Id="BPR16">20160126</element>
                </segment>
                <segment Id="TRN">
                    <element Id="TRN01">1</element>
                    <element Id="TRN02">883879217</element>
                    <element Id="TRN03">1205296137</element>
                </segment>
                <segment Id="REF">
                    <element Id="REF01">EV</element>
                    <element Id="REF02">1926706</element>
                </segment>
                <segment Id="DTM">
                    <element Id="DTM01">405</element>
                    <element Id="DTM02">20160125</element>
```

Source: Reprinted with permission by CentraMed/Hoap Health.

Figure 6.5 is a user-friendly translation generated from the raw XML data. As the reader can see, the information can now be used to uncover hidden problems, highlight trends, and improve cash flow.

■ Figure 6.5

User-friendly translation of 835 ERA

Acc Number	Patient Name	Denial Amt $	Payer	Denial Code	Adj Code	HCPCS Code	Revenue Code	Remark Code	NPI	Status	Work Queue	Duplicate	View
			All	50		All	All	All	All	Unreview		All	6 Month

Accounts Found: 699 (Displaying top 500 results) Unreviewed Update Status

Account Number	Patient Name	Provider/NPI	Payer	Contract	Total Charge $	Total Payment $	Total Adjustment $	Total Denial $	Patient Responsibility
		1912099094	UH		12,641.40	121.18	0.00	12,071.40	20.91
		1912099094	UH		12,641.40	121.18	0.00	12,071.40	20.91
		1912099094	UH		12,641.40	121.18	0.00	12,071.40	20.91
		1912099094	UH		9,253.23	0.00	0.00	9,253.23	0.00
		1912099094	BC/BS		8,041.54	2,331.81	0.00	5,310.00	5,310.00
		1912099094	BC/BS		13,971.14	6,322.46	0.00	5,227.00	6,561.00
		1912099094	CAHABA		7,946.00	422.02	0.00	5,170.00	107.60
		1912099094	CAHABA		5,466.00	0.00	0.00	5,126.00	0.00
Grand Totals:					$2,261,439.38	$449,996.95	$403.66	$116,630.20	

Acc No: 8A800005750622   No of Rec: 2   Unreviewed   Update Status

	DOS	Rev Code	HCPCS Code	Units	Charge $	Payment $	Adjustment $	Denial $	Adj Code	Modifier	Den Code	Rem Code	Line Status
	10/17/2017	0636	J2357	90	12,071.40	0.00	0.00	12,071.40				PI-50	Unreviewed
	10/17/2017	0260	96372	2	$70.00	121.18	448.82	0.00	CO-253,PR-3,CO-45				Unreviewed
Grand Totals				93	$12,641.40	$121.18	$448.82	$12,071.40					

Source: Reprinted with Permission by CentraMed/Hoap Health.

Many payers or their contractors will send individual letters to the hospital, and they often float around the facility until they find their destination. This process can lead to delays and missed deadlines, thus serving as another reason that contract addendums are so important; the name of the specific designee to send these letters to—or, better still, the exact business office or revenue cycle team—should be clearly specified in the contract addendum. Except for the information maintained by the appeal team (based on our experience), there is rarely any finance report on denials, reasons for the denials, the physicians involved, the payer source, the actions taken, and the amount recovered. Yet, first-pass denial information is an excellent barometer of inefficiencies either in the information provided by the different hospital service areas or incorrect coding on the claim form.

Hospital finance officers or revenue cycle leaders who have access to user-friendly denial information should share the information with hospital leaders and medical staff to enlist everyone's support in preventing denials in the first place. Monthly or quarterly denial information should be shared at every UR committee meeting and sent to medical department chairpersons. The information should not be blinded, although admittedly this may be politically difficult in many hospitals. Remember, unless the auditor invokes *Transmittal 541*, just because the hospital gets a denial doesn't mean the physician's claim will be denied, and in reality it rarely is.

Physician-specific denial information

Physician-specific denial information tells the backstory about how payers are responding to physicians' clinical decisions regarding admission, continued stay, and use of resources. In a consolidated revenue cycle program, the UR team has access to the first notice of a pending denial that finds its way to the biller's desk. When the causes of the pending denials are within the scope of influence of UR specialists, case managers, or the CDI team, these individuals can reach out to the physician involved and offer assistance to resolve. In many hospitals, these pending clinical denials are quickly forwarded to a centralized appeals team whose job it is to do whatever has to be done to reverse the decision. Most of the technical denials simply need claim form correction before generating a new—and accurate—claim form. Clinical denials involve a more complex process often including forwarding medical records and letters defending the physician's practice decision, which are typically prepared by the team members and endorsed by the physician. These are the hidden costs of back-end fixes that some companies estimate at $118 to $750 per account.

Physicians may be more interested in a reminder of the effect that denials may have on their patients. Patients generally react when they find out, after reading their explanation of benefit notices, that nothing was paid to the hospital. Calls to the billing office from these patients are commonplace, according to many PFS directors, and it falls to the billing office personnel to explain why the hospital did not get paid. All in all, it can be a public relations nightmare, although it is gratifying that patients will make these calls even when the patient themselves cannot be held responsible for the costs.

Armed with physician-specific denial information and the support of the medical leadership, case managers, UR specialists, and CDI teams can target their efforts to the neediest physicians. For example, if the data shows that Dr. Smith's heart failure cases are routinely denied due to inadequate documentation justifying an inpatient admission (CARC 150 on the list provided earlier in the chapter), then a member of the team should proactively engage Dr. Smith when he next admits a heart failure patient. Team members can use this data to help Dr. Smith understand the importance of providing the right care at the right time in the right place, and they are not casting any judgment—they're just using the facts. Because payers are narrowing physician panels, Dr. Smith needs to know that this data may be used to remove him from a payer panel if his denials habitually demonstrate practices that vary widely from those of his peer group. In addition, complete and thorough documentation leads to more accurate measures of the physician's acuity, which leads to more accurate measurement for the many quality payment and public reporting programs. Physician-specific information is an incredibly valuable resource if the board and executives are committed to streamlining progression of care, reducing costs, and improving efficiency outcomes. Furthermore, most physicians are willing to help; they understand that the hospital is their office and that if the hospital can't pay its bills, or purchase new equipment, or spruce up the patient rooms, they no longer have a place to work. Even hospitalists, who are in high demand, want to put down roots to raise a family and want the local hospital to thrive.

Creating physician-specific denial reports from the EDI 835 is doable once the XML data is translated into usable information. But an internally prepared report serves the purpose as well. Figure 6.6 is a sample of a physician denial report that was presented at a UR committee meeting in a Midwest community hospital. The report was created by the appeals team, which tracked all clinical denials. When first introduced, the physicians were dubious about the accuracy of the data and challenged the UR department director. At the following UR committee meeting, which increased in physician attendance, the manager of the PFS office presented a slideshow that tracked the UR process of a few sample cases and included actual copies of the remittances and final denial letters received for several accounts, giving the physicians in attendance primary evidence of revenue that was billed but not received. The physician response was exceptionally positive, and the number one question among the physicians who were there was: "Why weren't we told about this before?"

That question is routinely asked, and we do not have a good answer. Yet, in our collective experience, we know firsthand that physicians want objective information pertaining to their patients or their practice. Yes, they will push back at first, which is why it is so important that all data presented at UR committee meetings must be carefully vetted to withstand the challenges.

■ **Figure 6.6**

Total denials after failed appeal: Physician list 1/1/2019 to 12/31/2019									
Physician	Total Dischgs	Lack of Med Necessity	Delay in proc or test	Outpt/Amb Surg	Delay in Disch	Converted to OBS	No preauth/ late notice	ALC/SNF Rate	Total Dollars Denied
Adler, Step	71		3						6,332
Ahmed, Al	168	28	6			5	2		301,771
Altamura, M	174	1							2,830
Altman, Jerold	49	4							5,892
Ambrose, G	76					8	4		35,862
Amin, Sama	20	3							1,930
Ammon, Serge	79	3							4,590
Appel, S	154	39				9			365,070
Aro, Dom D	28	9				2	3		116,733
Artuso,Levi	172	16		2		3			163,445
Asprinio, Dav	291	10	4			4			101,884
Axelrod, Gre	312	25	23		1			1	896,772
Babu, Ram P	28		4						4,170
Babu, Maya	44	8	8	3	1		9		26,075
Belkin, Beth M	72	1							2,340
Belkin, Rob N	132	2	5						14,580
Bennett, R	128	1					2		2,840
Benzil, Lo	44	18	1		6	4			38,661
Carosilla, Chr	39	4							17,220
Total	**2,081**	**172**	**54**	**5**	**8**	**35**	**20**	**1**	**2,108,997**

The appeal process

Every hospital manages the appeal process differently. Most technical/administrative denials are handled directly between the PFS biller and the responsible party: medical records, coding, ancillary service managers, et al. But when it comes to handling clinical denials, the best practice in our experience begins with identifying a central source to receive hard-copy or electronic remittance advices from the payers requesting additional information to process a claim. There are still some insurers that send these requests electronically, but many double-down and send hard copies. Read the contract or provider manual to confirm the process the payer uses and make sure it is one that is reasonable and practical. If the payer uses hard copies, make sure the contract addendum cites a name and department for the recipient. It is not uncommon for the appeal team to receive a letter that was hanging around the mail room for six months before someone decided to try to find the right slot to put it in. By the time the appeal team opens the letter, the time frame has expired and the claim is denied.

If the organization has a designated RAC coordinator, that role could be expanded to centrally coordinate all clinical appeal efforts. Some large hospitals have appeals teams dedicated entirely to coordinating all incoming notices and outgoing letters to avoid late submissions. Depending upon the size of the hospital and the denial experience, all denials may be forwarded to the appeals team, which will determine how to best process the appeal. Serving like an airport control tower, the appeals team will coordinate the activities required to respond to the denials. Claims not paid due to administrative or technical challenges (such as incorrect codes, wrong dates, etc.) are typically sent to the specific process owner for correction and response. Admission, level of care or discharge disputes, and other related quality issues may be managed by the team in conjunction with department representatives, including the UR office.

The Medicare appeal process is straightforward and features several levels. Each level request uses a standard form and, effective 8 July 2019, no longer has to be signed by the appellant (*Federal Register* 84 *FR* 19855):

- First level: Redetermination by MAC. New information can be introduced.
- Second level: Reconsideration by qualified independent contractor. New information can be introduced.
- Third level: Hearing by an administrative law judge. Office of Medicare Hearings and Appeals (OMHA). No new information can be introduced.
- Fourth level: Review by Medicare Appeals Council.
- Fifth level: Judicial review in U.S. District Court.

Commercial payer appeals, on the other hand, are fraught with frustration and fury. Generally, the appeal process varies based on the payer contract. Redeterminations or reconsiderations may be the first and/or last level of appeal open to the provider. A second-level appeal is usually peer-to-peer. The PA can earn his or her keep by being a successful negotiator in this arena, although the payer may demand to review with the attending physician rather than the PA or an external physician advisory service. A third-level appeal is very rare, but it is worth a try if new information surfaces. Back-end appeals will never disappear, but the total volume of denials and appeals should diminish once the hospital transforms from a back-end revenue cycle to a more effective front-end model.

References

American Hospital Association. (May 2020). Hospitals and health systems face unprecedented financial pressures due to COVID-19. Retrieved from *https://www.aha.org/guidesreports/2020-05-05-hospitals-and-health-systems-face-unprecedented-financial-pressures-due.*

American Hospital Association. (10 June 2021). UnitedHealthcare to delay new policy that would deny coverage for some ED visits. Retrieved from *https://www.aha.org/special-bulletin/2021-06-10-after-concerns-aha-and-others-unitedhealthcare-will-delay-new-policy.*

Beckham, J. (1996). Hearing the tidal wave. *Healthcare Forum Journal, 39*(2):68–72

CMS. (21 February 2020). State Operations Manual, Appendix A – Survey protocol, regulations and interpretive guidelines for hospitals. Retrieved from *https://www.cms.gov/Regulations-and-Guidance/Guidance/Manuals/downloads/som107ap_a_hospitals.pdf.*

CMSA. (2019). The practice of hospital case management: A white paper. Little Rock, AR.

Fakler, J., Ozkurtul, O., and Josten, C. (2014). Retrospective analysis of incidental non-trauma associated findings in severely injured patients identified by whole-body spiral CT scans. *Patient Safety in Surgery.* Retrieved from *https://pssjournal.biomedcentral.com/articles/10.1186/s13037-014-0036-3.*

Noor, P. (12 February 2020). Can we trust AI not to further embed racial bias and prejudice? Retrieved from *https://www.bmj.com/content/368/bmj.m363.*

Revenue cycle denials index. (2020). Change Healthcare LLC. Retrieved from *https://www.ache.org/-/ media/ache/about-ache/corporate-partners/the_change_healthcare_2020-revenue_cycle_denials_index. pdf.*

Ugarte Hopkins, J. B. (2021). Deconstructing the Concept of Condition Code 44. Retrieved from *https:// racmonitor.com/deconstructing-the-concept-of-condition-code-44/.*

Walton, M. (1986). *The Deming Management Method.* New York, Perigee Books.

CHAPTER 7

The Utilization Review Committee

Background Information

Before the turn of the century, Florence Nightingale had pioneered techniques for assessing and improving the quality of medical services and spurred advances in the training of nurses. Ernest Codman, a Boston surgeon, developed techniques to audit medical care and identify corrective strategies for treatment deficiencies. And in 1954, Fred Carter, a physician, wrote, "Why not appoint a standing hospital staff committee designated as the 'hospital utilization committee, to do in the field of hospital and medical economics what the tissue committee does . . . in the field of surgery. Abuses in the use of hospital services and facilities coming to the attention of this hospital utilization committee could be disciplined to the point of near deletion" (London, 1965).

Hospitals accepting Medicare and Medicaid payment must create a utilization review (UR) committee to review the medical necessity and appropriateness of admissions to the facility, duration of stay, and the professional services rendered, according to the *Conditions of Participation* (*CoP*) as spelled out in 42 *CFR* 482.30. While the *CoP* still use the terminology "UR committee," it is more common now to see a designation that reflects its broadened oversight, such as "utilization management," "resource management committee," or even "quality resource committee." For the purposes of this book, however, we shall accede to the *CoP* and use the designation "UR committee." Although all hospitals have a UR committee, not every hospital has a fully functional and effective UR committee. That distinction is a product of history, culture, and corporate courage.

When first convened back in the days following the creation of Medicare and Medicaid, the UR committee primarily consisted of a few physicians performing retrospective chart reviews of cases representing a percentage of all admissions or selected populations. The director of UR would roll in a cart stuffed with medical records—yes, paper records before electronic health records existed—and the few doctors at the committee meeting would review long-stay cases, short-stay cases, specific diagnoses, and questionable cases. In many hospitals, the UR director would also present tables of data, indicating the average length of stay, the number of outlier admissions, the number of condition code 44 changes, and, if available, data on denials. The more progressive UR committees, which were willing to face the wrath of the medical staff, would go one step further. In those hospitals, the questionable cases would be brought to the attention of the attending physician, who was asked to either provide additional information or to appear at the next

UR committee meeting to justify medical decisions. Because this information request was part of the committee's duties, it was included in the committee minutes, the offending physician was advised on findings, and life went on. Although many hospitals reported an improvement in documentation and length of stay as a result of the UR committee's educational work with the physicians, many physicians resented being questioned about their medical judgment, and UR committee members complained about the time it took away from their practice.

The work of the UR committee

Over the years, and in too many hospitals, the work of the UR committee became a perfunctory process. For many in hospital administration, the UR committee was a tool used to whitewash the behaviors of errant physicians and to meet the requirements of the UR *CoP* with a minimal amount of work and disruption. Although physicians kept the beds filled and contributed to the hospital's bottom line in a cost-based reimbursement era, administrators did little to prop up the committee's work. However, when the hospital industry moved from cost-based reimbursement to a prospective payment system in 1983, a renewed interest in the work of the UR committee surfaced, and the committee transcended its original chart review activities. Today, with hospitals undergoing transformation from a volume- to a value-based payment environment, further adjustments are taking place. Individual cases may still be brought to the attention of the UR committee, but the previous "bad apple" approach, which used retrospective chart review to target errant physicians or practices, segued into the use of analytics to monitor the appropriate use of the facility and services. Today, a casual review of UR plans from academic medical centers to small critical access hospitals (CAH) shows similar, well-defined functions of the UR committee, which include the following:

1. Develop a process for educating interns, residents, hospitalists, and members of the medical community regarding regulatory and UR issues

2. Identify actions and follow-up to improve utilization of hospital resources

3. Review cases reasonably assumed to be outliers, as determined by extended lengths of stay or extraordinarily high costs

4. Review data to identify potential utilization concerns involving members of the medical staff

5. Identify unwarranted variation in medical performance and quantify its dollar impact on the organization

6. Reviewing resource utilization data applicable to all patients regardless of payment source

7. Provide a forum to review resource utilization by diagnoses, departments, procedures, and/or practitioners with identified or suspected resource utilization issues

8. Review and approve resource utilization benchmarks or targets based on the recommendations of the appropriate specialties or professional societies

9. Identify how much hospital utilization trends differ from expected benchmarks and best practice recommendations by professional organization

10. Use transparent, risk-adjusted metrics to analyze patterns of practitioner or institutional care for selected patient populations

11. Consider and make recommendations on all matters related to the utilization of the hospital facility and its resources

Today, hospital UR committees are in a state of transition as healthcare reform has increased both regulatory and financial pressures on hospitals. UR committees have changed from predominantly chart review forums to data-rich analytical groups, from subcommittees of the medical staff to joint committees of the medical staff and the board of directors, and from a narrow membership of two or more attending physicians to a broad representation of medical service leaders who influence "admissions to the facility, the duration of stays, and the professional services rendered" (42 *CFR* §482.30).

Because today's UR committees benefit from data-rich outcomes, the work of the committee primarily focuses on review of trends and patterns concerning admissions, continued stay, and certain professional services. Based on its own review of data or referral from another source, the UR committee determines that a physician appears to be engaging in a pattern of unnecessary admissions, inappropriate use of outpatient/observation services, excessive duration of stays, or professional services other than the medical necessity of procedures and diagnostic tests. In these cases, the UR committee has several options to consider: a letter of guidance or education; collegial intervention often arranged by the physician advisor (PA), or in the absence of a PA, the physician's department chair; or working with someone, such as the PA, admission review specialist (ARS), or UR specialist who may be able to help the physician learn how to better manage utilization issues.

The UR committee has no formal authority, so in cases where the physician continues to engage in a pattern of inappropriate utilization despite the UR committee's efforts at intervention, it may refer the physician for review under the Ongoing Professional Practice Evaluation committee or the appropriate medical staff committee for review and possible action.

Forces behind the value of UR committee work

Reducing healthcare costs so they are more in line with the level of general inflation would appear to demand radical changes in the American healthcare industry. This would mean either major restructuring of the financing and delivery systems or major cutbacks through large shifts in costs to patients, severe limitation on patients' choices of hospital and physicians, and explicit rationing of some technologies for all or some individuals, or a combination of some or all of these. Society may not be willing to make such changes, particularly in the short run, and may opt instead for more moderate strategies to control healthcare expenditures. UR is one such strategy.

It is an unfortunate reality, however, that most cost containment strategies eventually disappoint both providers and recipients of healthcare services. Even when these strategies seem to reduce costs initially, trend projections do not appear to show an appreciably lower increase in total costs over the longer term. Given the effort and optimism it generally takes to commit a corporation which is paying the healthcare premiums for its employees, or a government, to a new program, it is not surprising that excessively high expectations often give way eventually to disillusionment. Unwarranted or excessive negativism can, in turn, be counterproductive and lead to premature abandonment of modest but still helpful strategies. The hospital's UR committee is one entity that has been impacted by these perceptions.

Nevertheless, the expanding body of regulations governing use of federal funds for healthcare contributes significantly to the changing composition and dynamics of the UR committee. The passage of the 2010 Patient Protection and Affordable Care Act introduced the most significant overhaul of CMS regulations in years, and the changes to the Inpatient Prospective Payment System, including the 2-midnight rule, broadened the scope of compliance issues that the UR committee must address. As a result, hospital UR committees are besieged with responsibilities much greater than originally envisioned, and they are struggling to find their place. To address these concerns and confirm the board's commitment to monitor the use of scarce resources, some hospitals are known to have aligned the UR committee with the medical staff's Ongoing Professional Practice Evaluation policies to clarify and support the UR committee efforts to use collegial and educational efforts to address resource utilization and performance issues.

Committee Membership

CMS' UR *CoP* include specific requirements for the composition of the UR committee, specifying that it must be composed of at least two doctors of medicine or osteopathy. The presence of "two or more practitioners" is an important component of the UR committee structure for a couple of reasons (42 *CFR* §482.30).

First, reviews may not be conducted by any individual who has a direct financial interest in the hospital or who was professionally involved in the care of the patient whose case is being reviewed. A physician on the committee who cares for hospitalized patients would need another UR committee member to review the case if they participated in the care of the patient during their hospital stay.

Second, determinations of the UR committee must be discussed with the practitioner responsible for the patient's care. If that practitioner disagrees with the determination of the first UR committee physician, a second committee physician must review it. Having at least two physician members on the UR committee allows these determinations to be made expeditiously when needed. Despite the "two or more practitioners" requirement, many small, rural hospitals are hard-pressed to find physicians willing to serve. In those cases, an outside group may be contracted, as long as that group has been approved by CMS as specified in 42 *CFR* §482.30.

Beyond the two physician member requirements, membership on the UR committee has expanded to address the full scope of committee responsibilities in all community hospitals and especially in teaching facilities, integrated delivery systems, and academic medical centers. Because the UR committee now looks at more than just admission and continuing stay appropriateness, committee participation has expanded beyond representatives of the medical and surgical staff. Today, members often include the following:

- *The director of emergency services:* The emergency department (ED) is the front door of the hospital and is where most admission decisions are made. As the gatekeeper for the majority of inpatient admissions, the medical director of emergency services is key to compliance with payer expectations of acute care medical necessity. The medical director of emergency services is not only responsible for the operations of the ED but also is in a position to influence the decisions of the emergency medicine physician and the admitting physician about hospitalizing patients and choosing the correct admission status.

- *The medical directors of laboratory and blood bank services, imaging, nuclear medicine, catheterization lab, and other hospital-sponsored programs:* These are directors who affect resource use and provide input on issues of utilization and medical necessity. The directors of these diagnostic and special service areas are beginning to feel resource utilization pressures, especially in light of the Medicare spending per beneficiary (MSPB) metric. Under the MSPB indicator, use of the services offered by these areas are under close scrutiny for medical necessity. Additionally, resource use per case is an important component in every at-risk contract where shared savings may be jeopardized if total resource utilization across the continuum exceeds contractual benchmarks. It is especially problematic in hospitals or accountable care organizations (ACO) that are experimenting with capitated rates or down-side risk contracts. The availability of services provided by these departments is also a crucial factor in ensuring that hospital patients receive necessary services on a timely basis, especially in this environment where moving the patient efficiently through the continuum of care is crucial to optimize the total cost of care.

- *Representatives of the hospital's nursing, case management, quality, revenue cycle/revenue integrity, and compliance leadership:* These individuals hold collective accountability for UR across their hospital departments, and therefore workforce members from each of these areas may offer valuable expertise to the committee. For example, the chief compliance officer is the source of policies and regulations governing hospital operations, nursing and case management offer the perspective of day-to-day patient flow and treatment appropriateness, and quality can inform and clarify the myriad private and governmental agencies that are evaluating and publishing hospital performance outcomes. This broad representation is crucial to provide a balanced view of all issues. For example, finance representatives may view an increase in observation stays as an issue that needs to be fixed, while the compliance officer can provide the perspective that the goal should be to ensure that every patient be placed in the proper status, regardless of the reimbursement.

- *Members of the hospital's board of directors:* The board of directors is the fiduciary of all the hospital's resources and serves on behalf of the community; as such, the board works to ensure that the organization's resources are used in a reasonable, appropriate, and legally accountable manner. The presence of a board representative at the hospital's UR committee meeting is more common today than ever before. These board members also play another crucial role: ensuring that the full board is aware of the work of the UR committee and that no single physician or group of physicians can bypass the important work of the UR committee by approaching hospital leadership or board members and asking for help in "calling off 'those people' who keep telling me what to do and trying to throw my patients out of the hospital."

Reporting structure

UR committees are subcommittees of the medical staff, but because UR's focus shifted from individual peer/chart review to review of resource utilization trends and patterns, there are committees that are more closely aligned with the fiduciary responsibilities of the board of directors as well as the medical staff. As a result, it's not unusual these days to see a member of the board sitting as a member of the UR committee. The *CoP* allow the UR committee to be categorized as one of the following:

- A staff committee of the institution
- A committee established by the local medical society and some or all of the hospitals in the locality
- A committee established in a manner approved by CMS

These last two options work best in small hospitals, such as CAHs, where it may be difficult to find two physicians willing to contribute their time to fulfill the UR responsibilities. Nevertheless, as the board's governance accountability increases beyond financial responsibilities—and to detract from any cynics who might otherwise perceive the UR committee as only financially driven—it's probably best to position the UR committee under the board's quality improvement committee, which is generally a joint committee of the board and medical staff. Doing so may help ensure that hospital leadership is taking clear, appropriate measures to provide the safest healthcare in the most efficient and effective manner. However organized, the intent is to bring utilization issues to the timely attention of the board without going through the multiple layers of bureaucratic review typical of many medical staff bylaws.

Hospital UR committees have no disciplinary power and depending upon your view, that could be a positive or detract from its influence. But as a neutral committee, it could wield influence on physician practice without being seen as punitive, though its findings and recommendations eventually flow into the Ongoing Professional Practice Evaluation (OPPE), medical departments, medical executive committee, and ultimately into the credentialing processes. When The Joint Commission introduced the OPPE standard in 2008, it effectively raised the bar on evaluating physician competency. Physicians are recredentialed every two years, and the credentialing committee of the medical staff must demonstrate that objective metrics reflecting the performance of the physician are evaluated on an ongoing basis to identify trends and patterns that could adversely affect patient outcomes as part of their recommendations to the board pertaining to renewing privileges. The metrics, which each hospital can develop, generally reflect patient care, safety, quality, and administrative outcomes, often couched as "good citizenship" metrics. The requirement that the evaluation process be ongoing was a dramatic change from the previous process, which typically occurred once every two years. The OPPE program is intended to be a means of evaluating professional performance on an ongoing basis for the following reasons:

- As part of the effort to monitor professional competency
- To identify areas for possible performance improvement by individual practitioners
- To use objective data in decisions regarding continuance of practice privileges

Utilization Review Plan

There is no single best practice format for the design of a UR plan. However, the most effective plans are streamlined, include the salient points that are required as cited in the CoP, and avoid detailed complexities (see Figure 7.1).

The plan must include the following:

- Broad scope of intended UR objectives
- The composition of the UR committee as specified in the *CoP*
- The inclusion of the PA and nonmedical staff advisors
- The functions of the committee
- What authority has been delegated to the committee and by whom
- Meeting content and review process
- Committee responsibilities
- The feedback loop to the C-suite, medical executive committee, the medical staff, quality staff, and the board of directors
- Approval of nationally recognized guidelines for first-level reviews if used
- Information about the ongoing review, revision, and approval of the plan

The *CoP* do not tell the facility how to carry out its UR responsibilities, but they provide guidance on what must be done. Each hospital must develop its own plan that meets regulatory requirements and reflects the culture and customs of the organization. Responsibility for compliance with CMS' UR requirements rests squarely on the hospital and how well it follows its own plan. Therefore, the plan should contain only the essential components, without extraneous content that could be used to cite the hospital for noncompliance *Key* with its own policies (such as setting specific rules for the number of charts reviewed or any scoring system used during first-level chart reviews).

The plan must include a brief snapshot of the processes used for admission, continuing stay, and resource utilization, all of which should be clearly defined but not overly specific. The details are best reserved for policies and procedures governing the UR program. The UR plan should contain properties that characterize each category of review rather than step-by-step details. For example, the category of pre-admission medical necessity review for a transfer request could be stated as follows:

> *Transfers: Agreement to accept a patient in transfer from another facility requires the approval of a hospital physician in advance of the transfer. Following review of medical documentation provided by the transferring hospital related to the patient's history, current clinical status, and proposed treatment plan, the accepting physician will confirm that the patient requires care that is not available at the transferring facility, and the hospital has the capability and capacity to provide necessary care. An agreement confirming that the patient, once stabilized and no longer requiring the higher level of care, will be transferred back to their original facility will be signed as part of the transfer process.*

■ **Figure 7.1**

Sample utilization review plan language

The hospital, its governing board, and its medical staff, in conformity with the requirements of the CMS, the state department of health, and other payers, do hereby define and describe its concurrent and continuous plan for the utilization of its facilities and services by those availing themselves of the hospital's services regardless of the source of payment.

Purpose of the plan: The general aim of this plan is to codify the obligations of the utilization review (UR) committee, the hospital, its medical staff, and its associates to advance evidence-based, high-quality, cost-effective, and safe care to our patients and our community.

Responsibility: The UR committee is responsible for identifying and addressing unusual patterns of care that do not meet standards for best practice or quality of care or that are outside the organization's endorsed benchmarks. Information pertinent to maintaining the quality, cost effectiveness, and safety of care will be shared with the medical staff via division chairs and the medical executive committee. Ultimate responsibility for safe care for all patients who are treated in this hospital rests with the governing board. The specific responsibility for monitoring resource utilization of the facility and services is delegated to the chief executive officer and the president of the medical staff, with the assistance of other designated personnel as listed under the organization and composition of the committee.

Organization and composition of the committee: The UR committee is composed of the physician advisor (who will serve as the UR committee chairperson), medical department chairpersons, the chief operating officer, and physicians and/or non-physician members to represent departments including utilization review, nursing, quality, compliance, pharmacy, laboratory, diagnostic imaging, respiratory, and finance. A member of the board serves as an ex-officio delegate to the committee. No person on the committee (or on a committee performing functions delegated by the UR committee) may have a financial interest in the hospital. No person may participate in the case review of any care in which he or she was professionally involved in providing care.

Sample utilization review plan language (cont.)

Authority: The UR committee has the authority to perform prospective, concurrent, or retrospective review of the medical record of any patient admitted to the hospital or treated on an outpatient basis; to review documents certifying medical necessity for acute care admission; to review resource utilization data to evaluate service line and/or physician performance; and to discuss findings with the physician or physicians concerned, but does not have the authority to take disciplinary action. Findings and recommendations of the UR committee are reported to the president of the medical staff, board of directors, and chief executive officer, who have the authority and responsibility for considering and acting on them.

Functions: The utilization review committee functions to do the following:

- Advance the practice of evidence-based care

- Promote cost-efficient utilization of hospital resources and services in accordance with the patient's acute medical needs and preferences

- Provide educational opportunities to engage the medical staff and hospital associates in efforts to demonstrate superior resource

- Identify and correct patterns of care and situational factors that may contribute to under-, over-, and/or inappropriate utilization of hospital resources and services

- Use objective data to assess physician practice trends and patterns regarding length of stay and resource utilization for the purpose of improving quality of care and service delivery

- Recommend and/or take corrective actions to improve resource utilization and the quality of care

Source: Stefani Daniels, RN, MSNA, ACM, CMAC, president and managing partner at Phoenix Medical Management, Inc., in Pompano Beach, Florida. Reprinted with permission.

The Wickline decision

From the physician's point of view, many UR specialists are intruding into clinical practice in a way that has a negative effect on quality of care by inappropriately mixing fiscal and medical treatment concerns. However, measures to manage the cost of care are necessary to reduce spiraling healthcare costs and to rein in avoidable expenses. Appropriately implemented, UR tries to balance the clinical needs of the patients with cost containment objectives. Nevertheless, there are some lessons to be learned about how rigorously the process should be applied.

In the 1986 *Wickline v State of California* case, Lois Wickline sued the state alleging that the Medi-Cal state insurance program caused her to be discharged prematurely, which resulted in a leg amputation. She had vascular insufficiency in her legs and was admitted to undergo a major revascularization procedure. Medi-Cal approved a 10-day hospital stay. Due to a difficult recovery, her surgeon requested an additional eight days of acute care. The insurer approved only four days, and Mrs. Wickline was discharged at the end of those four days. Nine days later, she was readmitted with blood clots in the leg and an infection, which resulted in an amputation. She sued the insurance company, claiming that its UR process failed to approve an extension of her hospitalization and was the cause of her amputation.

The California Court of Appeals rejected her claim. However, in its opinion, the court implicitly criticized the physician for not advocating for his patient and strongly suggested that the physician should be liable for discharging her when he knew it was dangerous to do so, regardless of what the insurance company decided to do. The court wrote, "If, in his medical judgment, it was in his patient's best interest that she remain in the acute care hospital setting for an additional four days beyond the extended time period originally authorized by Medi-Cal, Dr. Polansky should have made some effort to keep Wickline there ... Medi-Cal was not a party to that medical decision and therefore cannot be held to share in the harm resulting if such decision was negligently made" (Brenner and Bal, 2009). The *Wickline v California* case is a seminal decision in the area of UR liability and is one of those cautionary tales we mentioned previously.

A UR decision invariably turns on whether a treatment or service is "medically necessary." Definitions of medical necessity vary greatly, but all seem to explicitly imply that it involves the exercise of good medical practice for the treatment of illness or injury. A determination of medical necessity is always a judgment call, and every reviewer must be careful not to apply an overly restrictive standard. This is the reason behind our position that while recognized guidelines are good tools, they do not replace the narrative documentation that should reflect the patient's condition that warrants hospitalization or continued stay. When those two components are not in synch, and the physician is reluctant to clarify his judgment call in writing, then the case should be brought to the attention of the PA. As discussed throughout this book, the UR staff and PA are tasked with ensuring that patients are not only receiving medically necessary care but that the care is provided in the right setting.

The Utilization Review Committee Agenda

One way to provide a consistent structure to conduct a UR committee meeting is to create a standard agenda for each meeting. Doing so can also help maximize productivity during the meeting so that everyone's time is used wisely. Experience has shown that when discussions stray from the topic, interest lags and attendance suffers. After the obligatory call to order, roll call, and approval or correction of the minutes of the previous meeting, a typical UR committee agenda may contain reports regarding the following:

1. Admission review: Raw and relational data on inpatient cases that did not present with adequate documentation of medical necessity and/or did not meet payer guidelines for inpatient admission.

2. Resource utilization: Divergence from best practice guidelines regarding imaging, lab, blood utilization, or other selected resources. Review of length of stay and cost per case for high-volume diagnoses.

3. Avoidable days/avoidable delays: Review of this data can lead to discussion/actions among committee members to fix common bottlenecks, such as availability of services on weekends, rounding too late to discharge patients, ordering "while you are here" tests, difficulty in transferring patients to certain skilled nursing facilities off hours, etc.

4. Antibiotic stewardship: Divergence from best practice and formulary guidelines.

5. Evidence-based care: Experiential data on the appropriate use or variations from medical staff-endorsed guidelines, protocols, and order sets.

6. Payer denials: Electronic remittance advice (835 notifications) for first-pass experience and post-appeal outcomes.

7. Documentation integrity results: The activities of the clinical documentation integrity (CDI) team and the physician's response to queries.

8. Outlier cases: Review of selected extended-stay, high-cost cases.

9. UR committee interventions: The activities of the PA on behalf of the committee, such as condition code 44 and postdischarge self-denials.

10. Old business covered by the UR committee: This may include the following:

    a. Questions or actions that were pending at the last session

    b. Any unfinished business that did not come up at the last session

    c. Anything from the last session that was not completed

11. New business covered by the UR committee: This may include new resource utilization projects or regulatory updates and would also include highlights from the most recent payment reports received by the hospital from CMS, such as the following:

    a. Program for Evaluating Payment Patterns Electronic Report (PEPPER): We previously mentioned PEPPER, the comparative data report that provides hospital-specific Medicare data statistics for discharges vulnerable to improper payments. By distributing this report to hospitals, with similar data available to the QIOs and all Medicare contractors, CMS hopes to encourage hospital leaders to target high-risk payment error areas, such as billing, coding, and admission necessity issues, for internal audits. PEPPER uses hospital-specific claims data to compare one facility to similar Medicare providers in these risk areas. PEPPER is an underutilized comparative report but is a valuable resource for revenue cycle teams, UR committees, and compliance officers. We urge readers to get a copy of their hospital's PEPPER, learn how to read the data, and become a proponent of monitoring high-risk areas. PEPPER information can be found at *https://pepper.cbrpepper.org/*.

    b. Comparative Billing Reports (CBR): A CBR provides comparative billing data for an individual healthcare provider. The reports contain tables and graphs created from real data with an explanation of findings that compare provider's billing and payment patterns to those of their peers on both a national and state level. CBR study topic(s) are selected because they are prone to improper payments. For health systems that employ physicians, CBRs are crucial to determine if the physician's coding requires further attention. For additional information and examples of CBRs, visit *https://cbrpepper.org/*.

12. Announcements: Any announcements must be made before the meeting is adjourned and may include discussion about new staff resources or planned education and training programs offered to hospital associates or the medical staff.

Outcomes

Within each agenda item is the opportunity to demonstrate the outcomes of the work of UR specialists. For example, item 1, admission reviews, isn't on the agenda simply to state the volume of reviews performed during the last reporting period. Rather, the topic is an opportunity to demonstrate the influence of the UR specialist on the physician to place the patient in the correct status based on guidelines and documentation. The report discussed during the meeting may cite, for example, that of the 438 ED patients initially targeted for inpatient hospitalization, 53 cases were successfully placed in observation or referred to a more appropriate community resource through the influence of the ARS. Each of those pieces of data can then be quantified in some manner (e.g., average revenue per patient day) to demonstrate the financial impact.

Similarly, item 2, resource utilization, can target a specific resource being monitored by the UR team within a given time period. For example, a recent study demonstrated that compared with patients treated by other hospitalists, the patients of high-consulting hospitalists had longer lengths of stay and were less likely to go home, and there was no significant difference in their mortality at 30 days or their likelihood of all-cause readmission. This may prompt monitoring of the volume of questionable consults generated by the hospitalists (e.g., cardiac consult for a noncardiac admission diagnosis) (Stevens et al., 2020).

Efforts to measure outcomes don't always begin with perfect measures, but fortunately the fastest way to improve outcome measures is to start using them. We recall that the current state-of-the-art measures used for cardiac surgery were originally motivated by public reporting of very rudimentary (and, some thought, misleading) mortality data. But in response, the Society of Thoracic Surgeons began developing measures that have become far more sophisticated, are applied to a much wider array of surgeries, and are driving improvement nationwide.

Data Support

Approximately 18% of the U.S. gross domestic product (GDP) is spent on healthcare, and the current state of resource utilization has much room for improvement. The GDP is the total of all the goods and services produced in the U.S. in a given year, so in the simplest terms, approximately 18 cents of every dollar generated in the U.S. is spent on healthcare. If 18 cents are spent on healthcare, what is left to spend on other necessities? To put these numbers in historical perspective, back in 1965 when Medicare and Medicaid were created, healthcare consumed less than 6% of the U.S. GDP.

Every single administration since Nixon, who was the first to describe the unsustainable growth in healthcare costs as a crisis, has promised, in one form or another, to cut costs and improve quality. But it is difficult to pursue lower costs and good stewardship of resources unless the healthcare industry provides good data to identify where overutilization or underutilization occurs. Accurate data—data that are vetted for computational accuracy—are essential to manage, integrate, interpret, share, and present information to a broad range of care providers.

But when working with physicians, using data to build consistency around a goal is fraught with challenges. Speaking about a physician's performance based on metrics can be like walking into a hornet's nest. Physicians will often challenge data, and rarely do they blindly accept negative data about their own performance. They are likely to become defensive when presented with data that does not mesh with how they see themselves. In addition, physicians commonly believe that their own practice is different from the norm in that their patients are older or sicker or more complicated in general. Therefore, the UR committee must have access to a dedicated analyst to collect credible, useful data that can hold up to the inevitable pushback from physicians. The critical importance of data was cited by the National Academy of Medicine as being "foundational to the concept of a learning health system—one that leverages and shares data to learn from every patient experience, and feeds the results back to clinicians, patients and families, and health care executives to transform health, health care, and health equity" (National Academy of Medicine, 2020).

In addition, physicians must be taught a new statistical model for performance improvement. Although physicians are generally familiar with the statistical models used in clinical trials and controlled research projects, the performance improvement approach is quite different. In the improvement models originally conceived by W. Edwards Deming and Walter A. Shewhart, a cycle of improvement (Plan, Do, Check, Act) was used to analyze, measure, and identify sources of process variations that compromise outcomes.

Deming argued that every service has multiple key quality characteristics. To improve outcomes, one must identify the process attributes that create those characteristics. This type of data collection involves nothing more than planning for and obtaining useful information on key quality characteristics created through operational and practice processes. The results raise questions that need to be addressed to further understand and reduce unintended outcomes and establish a factual basis for making decisions.

Data will serve as benchmarks by which the medical staff can continuously measure and compare their practice performance both internally and externally. In preparation for transitioning a UR committee from a largely case review approach to a data-driven model to objectively identify and target performance and resource management improvement projects, consider the following strategies.

Solicit input from those who will be receiving the data to identify measures that directly indicate the success of any change effort. For example, in 2016, the AABB (formerly the American Association of Blood Banks) published new recommendations for evaluating red blood cell transfusions. Previously, physicians would sometimes view asymptomatic patients with a hemoglobin threshold of 9–10 g/dL as anemic and in need of a transfusion. The new guidelines strongly recommend adherence to a "restrictive transfusion threshold of 7 g/dL for hospitalized adult patients who are hemodynamically stable, including critically ill patients," and 8 g/dL for "patients undergoing orthopedic surgery, cardiac surgery and those with preexisting cardiovascular disease" (Carson et al., 2016). To reduce unnecessary transfusions, the UR committee should seek consensus about using this guideline to drive change, and a data analyst should work with the committee to produce data on the hospital's current status (see Figures 7.2 and 7.3).

■ **Figure 7.2**

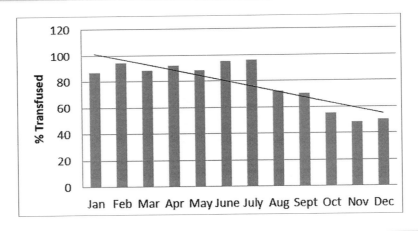

Transfusion with a hemoglobin threshold greater than 7 g/dL: Change over time

Source: Stefani Daniels, RN, MSNA, ACM, CMAC, founder and senior advisor at Phoenix Medical Management, Inc., in Pompano Beach, Florida. Reprinted with permission.

■ Figure 7.3

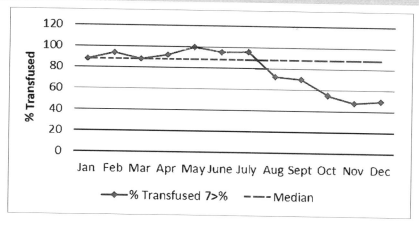

Transfusion with a hemoglobin threshold greater than 7 g/dL: Statistical evidence of change

Source: Stefani Daniels, RN, MSNA, ACM, CMAC, founder and senior advisor at Phoenix Medical Management, Inc., in Pompano Beach, Florida. Reprinted with permission.

Choose data displays wisely to ensure they tell the best story to drive improvement. For example, using the displays presented in Figures 7.2 and 7.3, compare a typical bar graph to a run chart. The bar graph shows change over time, but the run chart more clearly demonstrates statistical evidence of a change, as seen in the sequence of seven consecutive points above the median from January through August. This pattern would not appear randomly, so something must have happened in August to precipitate such a significant drop in transfusions. Although both graphs will raise some productive dialogue, the run charts are especially useful: they "are one of the most important tools for assessing the effectiveness of change" (Institute for Healthcare Improvement, 2015).

Meaningful data means that the data is actionable; one can peruse the information, easily decipher the patterns and trends over time, and take action based on the findings. The reports in Figures 7.2 and 7.3 provide an overview of the change over time in the use of blood transfusions in patients with hemoglobin greater than 7 g/dL. These graphs show a reduced number of transfusions starting in August, when the lab began its educational campaign. Nevertheless, the UR committee determines that the current 50% rate is still too high. Although they continue the educational campaign, they ask the data analyst to present comparative, physician-specific data. If the committee believes that this project is important enough to measure, then it should provide transparent feedback to each physician (see Figure 7.4). Physicians are highly competitive and have a strong desire to succeed. The UR committee chairperson can use these traits to leverage improvement efforts; therefore, using blind data and obscuring individual physician identities will negate the positive effects of peer pressure. Over time, as physicians become accustomed to the committee's new way of doing things, sharing results can become a powerful motivator.

■ Figure 7.4

Checklist for sharing utilization review committee resource reports

✓ Measurement and feedback are critical supports to drive change in resource utilization.

✓ The information must be shared in a way that is easily understandable and useful.

✓ The information must be presented so that it is actionable. Actionable data enables the receiver to do something with the findings. It answers not just what, but where, when, or why and can be used for decisions, to stimulate problem-solving discussions, and to provide context to ensure strategic alignment with organizational goals.

✓ The information must be unblinded and drive resource utilization improvement.

✓ Raw data on volumes or productivity has no place at the UR committee. How many patients were admitted, how many cases were reviewed, how many times condition code 44 was used, and how much the hospital lost to payer denials are not actionable data. Although each of these metrics may be of interest to some committee members, they should be translated into more appropriate utilization projects.

Once the UR committee is fully functioning as the major force within the hospital and among the medical staff for reducing inappropriate utilization of the facility and services, it must work out a process for holding physicians accountable for improvement. The UR committee can provide many forms of positive support to drive change, but not all individuals will succeed. When performance does not improve, there must be consequences. The UR committee has no disciplinary authority, but it can recommend an appearance before the medical executive committee, a talk with the board, peer-to-peer coaching, attendance at an education program, referral to OPPE, or limitation of hospital privileges. Set clear expectations; otherwise, the committee sends a message that monitoring resource utilization is optional.

Resource Utilization

The *CoP* specifically cites that the UR committee must establish a mechanism to "review professional services provided, to determine medical necessity and to promote the most efficient use of available health facilities and services" [42 *CFR* §482.30 (c)(1)(iii)]. For our purposes, therefore, resource utilization refers to activities undertaken by the hospital's UR committee, and by extension, leaders whose responsibility it is to manage resources, to monitor, evaluate, and inform hospital associates on how costly resources are used in the care of hospitalized patients. Physicians make decisions about hospital resource allocation on a daily basis but rarely get any feedback on whether those resource were used appropriately.

The UR committee is the forum for reporting and mediating resource utilization information, and it can take steps to influence individual physician practice behaviors. Too often, however, physicians feel that their years of education and training mean that they can forgo oversight, and they may need encouragement via use of data and peer pressure to embrace UR committee recommendations. Most physicians will admit that they are often challenged by issues outside of direct patient care, such as in areas of throughput, rules and regulations, coding and documentation requirements, and quality reporting. Nevertheless, they must be convinced that their practice behaviors influence the bottom line for themselves, the organization, and their patients and that modifying those behaviors can mean improvements for all.

Physician-specific practice profiles

Even without the benefit of evidence-based guidelines, comparative physician-specific practice profiles demonstrate the physician's current practices regarding costs associated with resource utilization, length of stay (LOS), volume of consultants or diagnostic tests ordered, and other assorted indicators of effective practice. Many hospital executives regularly produce this information and share it with members of their medical staff, typically through the UR committee or the medical staff quality committee. Given the extent of data transparency, these executives—and the hospital boards supporting them—believe that sharing practice information is the best way to keep physicians informed of how the payers and regulators view them. They can also use this data to target improvement opportunities. At the other extreme are hospital leaders and boards who believe that shielding the medical staff from comparative data reports will mollify the physicians, who in turn will continue to admit patients. This latter tactic is doomed to failure. In the "good old days" when hospital admissions were not scrutinized at every step, these physicians did bring significant revenue. But going forward, we suspect that the care provided by the physician with poor documentation and lack of medical necessity is not going to be paid. It is the rare hospital with large endowments and alternative sources of revenue that can survive when the care they provide to patients results in denial after denial. It is a running joke among hospital finance people that even if they lose money on every admission, they make it up on volume.

Whatever approach is used in a hospital, know that objective, comparative physician practice profiles are excellent resources to identify practice patterns that may compromise progression of care, increase costs and risks, and jeopardize at-risk payment methodologies that depend upon quality metrics. Payers and ACOs are also using these profiles to narrow the panels of physicians available to their members.

For example, if a hospital is trying to identify best practice for the care of heart failure patients, it should produce a severity-adjusted report itemizing all of the all-patients refined diagnosis-related groups' (APR-DRG) 194 heart failure cases. Unlike the Medicare Severity-DRG (MS-DRG) system, APR-DRG includes all patients—not just Medicare patients—and expands the basic DRG structure by adding four severity categories to each DRG to demonstrate differences in severity of illness and risk of mortality.

Wide variations in patterns of practice within a single DRG generally indicate differences in resource utilization (as generally measured by cost). However, as research has shown, these differences do not necessarily correlate with quality of care. Using the resources cited on the claim form that are reported under physicians' national provider identifier (NPI) numbers, the analytic team will organize those cases according to units of resource utilization or according to the costs of those resources, ranging from those who use less than their peer group average to those who use more than their peer group average (see Figure 7.5). The resources consumed by the average will probably be considered as representing best practice. The goal here is to work with the high outliers to see how their practice differs from the average practice, offer assistance to improve, and publicly acknowledge the lower-resource-use outliers who can set the standard for their colleagues.

If still using LOS as an evaluative metric, consider the source of the data and its statistical significance. Recall that GMLOS is derived from hundreds of thousands of patients, while the physician under review in your facility may only have one or two patients within one MS-DRG.

■ **Figure 7.5**

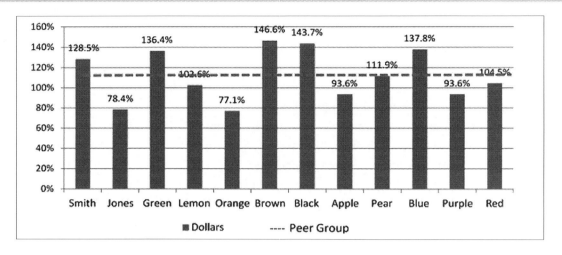

Source: Stefani Daniels, RN, MSNA, ACM, CMAC, founder and senior advisor at Phoenix Medical Management, Inc., in Pompano Beach, Florida. Reprinted with permission.

Often, the volume of consultants may be the culprit; hospitalists usually do not realize that the resources used by their consultants are currently assigned to the attending physician's NPI number. CMS is working on a project to assign attribution to the actual provider, but it is still in the planning phase. If an attending hospitalist calls in a cardiologist to treat his or her heart failure patient, any orders that the consultant may write will be attributed to the attending physician. Most hospitalists are unaware of this bit of coding trivia. Additional consultants typically equate to additional orders, which then results in more time spent in the hospital but does not necessarily result in better outcomes. According to an article in the February 2020 issue of *JAMA Network Open,* hospitalists who use more consultants than their peers do not have better mortality rates or fewer readmissions than their colleagues (Stevens, 2020). A high number of consultants also delays progression of care and timely transition, because the attending physician won't discharge a patient until each consultant agrees on the discharge. Unfortunately, nurses, case managers, or UR specialists often have the job of coordinating discharge agreements and medication reconciliation among the physicians.

Hospital leaders must try to keep a lid on healthcare costs to successfully manage upside or downside risk contracts. They must reinforce the value equation—that is, improving quality while keeping costs affordable. If a member of the medical staff has a confirmed pattern of misuse or excessive use of resources, this behavior must be discussed with the offending physician, and a nonconfrontational coach, such as a PA, may help push the physician toward quality improvement. A PA is best positioned to help the physician understand the role of the UR committee and the financial and safety implications of excessive or misused interventions.

For example, the PA might make rounds with the physician and provide real-time, one-on-one coaching involving both documentation advice and ways to best manage patients within evidence-based protocols. The PA may also involve others in this pursuit. For example, if the data objectively demonstrates that Dr. X has an ongoing pattern of overuse of CT scans, the PA can suggest that the chief radiologist reach out to Dr. X to clarify CT parameters.

The PA may also suggest that a case manager, UR specialist, or CDI specialist work with the physician to provide real-time coaching. Physicians may feel more comfortable working with a favorable colleague rather than a peer or supervisor who may be seen as threatening. The important thing to remember in those circumstances is that a nonmedical coach must avoid questioning medical judgment and limit coaching advice to practice decisions or documentation improvement. For example, diagnosing aspiration pneumonia is a product of medical judgment, whereas choosing which antibiotic to use among the many choices offered to the physician on the culture and sensitivity (C&S) report is a practice decision. The CDI specialist may coach the physician on the documentation needed to clinically validate the diagnosis of aspiration pneumonia without interfering with medical judgment. If the patient requires a specific antibiotic that may cost more than one listed on the C&S report, the CDI specialist can guide the physician as to what elements to document to support the decision to prescribe that antibiotic.

The CDI specialist, the UR specialist, and the PA can help the physician understand the importance of documentation in both supporting medical necessity and justifying what may appear to be higher-than-expected utilization. It is becoming more common to see reporting of observed versus expected data on costs, mortality, LOS, and many other measures. Physicians need to understand the influence their documentation has on those calculations as well as the impact that poor outcomes will have on their reputation, the hospital's reputation, and the financial viability of both. The MS-DRG and APR-DRG systems both have several levels of each diagnosis. When faced with data suggesting a physician has higher resource costs, longer length of stay, or higher mortality than others, it may not be a quality-of-care issue but rather a documentation issue. By simply documenting more specifically, the expected LOS or mortality rate can change significantly.

Hospitalists, UR, and resource utilization

As healthcare began its shift from inpatient to ambulatory services, the role of the hospitalist emerged as essential to manage the increasingly complex hospital patient. Gone are the days that most community physicians round on the patients. Instead, they've retreated to their office, and the job of caring for their hospitalized patients was left to hospitalists. Today, more than 60,000 hospitalists do the job for them (Wood, 2020). Since it emerged as a specialty in 1996, hospital medicine has transformed the care of inpatients. The hospital is the hospitalist's office—their place of business. And yet, they and their interns and resident colleagues have little if any knowledge about the business requirements that influence how their business operates and its impact on how they care for their patients. Indeed, among the most dissatisfying aspects of their job is the volume of rules and regulations (Wood, 2020).

On the other hand, we also have noted a new appreciation of the work of the UR specialist once the hospitalist is exposed to the countless complexities of the regulatory environment and marketplace expectations. The role of the PA in hospitals is rapidly expanding, and getting hospitalists involved on the UR committee is a first step that may lead to a part-time or even full-time role as a PA.

In addition, and at the expense of repeating ourselves, we urge the executive team to develop a formal onboarding program for hospitalists, medical students, interns, and residents to expose them to current topics in healthcare that impact the business of caring for their patients. Topics such as healthcare law, hospital operations, regulatory oversight, government policy, and information as basic as how hospitals get paid will meet the feedback and mentoring millennials seek. We know first-hand that young millennial physicians are especially receptive to coaching to help them be more efficient and more effective.

We believe that executive teams must do more to inform all hospital associates of the business pressures heaped upon hospitals over the past few decades. All hospitals want to offset the growing financial pressures they face by growing their market through attracting new patients and increasing the satisfaction of their existing patients. All hospitals play a role in meeting those goals but may not be adequately equipped to do so. Educating staff on the business of healthcare has been proven to be one of the most powerful tools at executives' disposal, because the staff can in turn educate their friends, neighbors, and relatives. Not long ago, we encountered a chief operating officer who held monthly informal lunch and learn sessions dedicated exclusively to the business aspects of operating a hospital. She reported that attendance began modestly, but she recently had to find a larger space to accommodate a standing-room-only audience of hospital associates from every department in the hospital.

Several years ago, one of the authors of this book taught a class in the Master of Science in Nursing program at the University of Pennsylvania. Some of the students were entry level and completely new to nursing, while other students were experienced practitioners. No matter the level of experience, most of the students were skeptical about the need to learn healthcare business concepts as they entered the course. By the end of the semester, they were able to make a business case on why it is essential for all clinicians to have a working knowledge of how hospitals operate and why understanding finance is essential to improving the quality of patient care. With change in hospital payment models hanging over the horizon and the need to preserve resources so they are available to the entire community, it's time for hospitalists, clinicians, and associates to acknowledge that their performance affects not only their patients' health but the financial health of their organization. And it's time that the C-suite recognizes the value of investing in staff education.

References

Brenner, L. H., and Bal, B. S. (June 2009). Patient care vs. economics: How liable are physicians and facilities in this environment. Orthopedics Today. Retrieved from *https://www.healio.com/news/orthopedics/20120325/patient-care-vs-economics-how-liable-are-physicians-and-facilities-in-this-environment.*

Carson, J. L., et. al. (2016). Red blood cell transfusion thresholds and storage. Journal of the American Medical Association. Retrieved from *https://www.ncbi.nlm.nih.gov/pubmed/27732721.*

Centers for Medicare & Medicaid Services. (n.d.). *Condition of Participation: Utilization Review.* 42 CFR 482.30.

Institute for Healthcare Improvement. (2015). Run Chart Tool. Retrieved from *http://www.ihi.org/resources/Pages/Tools/RunChart.aspx.*

London, M. (September 1965). Medical staff utilization committees. *Inquiry, 2*(2) p. 77–95. Retrieved from *http://www.jstor.org/stable/41348514.*

Whicher, D., Ahmed, M., Siddiqi, S., Adams, I., Grossmann, C., and Carman, K. (Eds.). (2020). Health Data Sharing to Support Better Outcomes. National Academy of Medicine. Retrieved from *https://nam.edu/wp-content/uploads/2020/11/Health-Data-Sharing-to-Support-Better-Outcomes_prepub-final.pdf.*

Stevens, J. P., Hatfield, L. A., et al. (21 February 2020). Association of Variation in Consultant Use Among Hospitalist Physicians With Outcomes Among Medicare Beneficiaries. *JAMA Network Open, 3*(2):e1921750. doi:10.1001/jamanetworkopen.2019.21750.

Wood, D. (2020). 15 Surprising Facts About Hospitalists. Staff Care: Locum Tenens Blog, March 5. Retrieved from *https://www.staffcare.com/physician-blogs/15-surprising-facts-about-hospitalists-in-2020/.*

CHAPTER 8

Leadership, Information, and Closing Comments

Information Is Knowledge

Value-based care (VBC) is a reimbursement model based on the quality of care rather than the quantity of care. When the physician is paid under fee-for-service models, payment is based on the quantity of services provided. In contrast, VBC is based on the overall effect that service has on the patient in terms of costs and quality. In other words, risk is shifted from the payer to the provider. For example, 67% of Humana's Medicare Advantage (MA) members are covered by some type of value-based payment model, from global capitation to fee-for-service with some shared savings (Holt, 2020). Value-based payment models have not yet attained the same penetration in hospitals as they have for physicians.

To survive in a VBC environment, success is dependent on how well the organization can track quality and expenses, identify opportunities to curb avoidable expenses and improve quality, and demonstrate the success of quality improvement and cost-saving activities. For each of these must-haves, information is essential to doing the job and doing it well.

Leadership and information

There are as many leadership theories as there are theorists. But it's fair to say that most utilization review (UR) specialists instinctively look to someone who guides the team and provides it with valuable information on the work that they do, the analytics they need, and the outcomes they generate.

Throughout this book, we have identified three kinds of information essential to the success of contemporary UR. The first is *environmental information,* which is defined as information from external sources often in the form of new statutes, organizational directives, or payer policies. The practice of UR is heavily influenced by statutory requirements that are generated by the federal or state governments and change frequently. Staying abreast of those changes is essential for organizational compliance and to protect against risk. The chief compliance officer is generally the key resource for the UR program leader in this area, as are members of the executive team or revenue cycle leadership. The UR program leader is then responsible for sharing the information with the UR team as well as other revenue cycle staff that work with UR. In addition, there must be a mechanism to share that information with members of the clinical team so they understand the rationale behind any changes in expectations. The classic case in point goes back to August 2013 when the 2-midnight rule was introduced and information on the rule was shared with medical leadership. Unfortunately, this information was not always presented with a clear explanation of the rule and the associated requirements, and as a consequence confusion continues to plague many hospitalist teams as new generations of physicians join them. We have attempted to give you resources that will help you navigate the regulatory environment, which plays such an important part in the world of the admission review specialist (ARS) and the UR specialist.

Data-generated information is generally created from various data sources and provides insight into how the organization is performing. Artificial intelligence, big data, and predictive analytics are indispensable tools that assess information in a way no single clinician could. If we mine and analyze large data sets, we can distill information for making better-informed decisions about patient care. These tools also help identify fraud, waste, and abuse. Unfortunately, many hospitals rarely have access to perfect information, and despite the explosion of electronic health records (EHR) and data warehouses, data-generated information is usually subject to considerable errors, or the hospital may not have the talent or the technology to translate the data into meaningful information. Nevertheless, if we acknowledge that the essential purpose of hospitalization is to improve the health of our patients, it is axiomatic that the board, the medical staff, and every hospital associate must be willing to measure the health results as well as the costs of delivering care for each patient to justify their existence. Through their travels to hospitals across the country, we have tried to give you examples of how hospital executives and program leaders use data to better meet the demands of the marketplace and improve the quality of care for their patients.

Knowledge management literature often points out that it is important to distinguish between data, information, and knowledge. The generally accepted view sees data as raw facts that become information as data is combined and given meaning, which subsequently becomes knowledge as meaningful information is put into context and used to make predictions. This view sees data as a prerequisite for information, and information as a prerequisite for knowledge. A prime example is the information on throughput delays and avoidable days as well as payer denials, which are elusive pieces of information in many hospitals and places the UR specialist in an untenable position. UR specialists are expected to make sure that the hospital gets paid but rarely have access to information that would tell them where the risk of not getting paid rests.

There is also the challenge of interoperability. Medical records do not flow seamlessly from one organization to another, and, therefore, data sharing processes are jeopardized. As we emerge from a crippling pandemic, the social distancing and isolation that affected us all bears a striking similarity to our healthcare information: siloed and disconnected. In the past, the healthcare industry has never been incentivized to share data. Leaders of healthcare organizations haven't wanted to share what they deem to be proprietary information with competitors who could use it to target high-value patients or gain insights into clinical or business practices. But rules from the Office of the National Coordinator for Health Information Technology and the Centers for Medicare & Medicaid Services (CMS) will force the adoption of an infrastructure that will give patients easier access to their own records and ensure that technology is able to gather and prepare data from disparate sources in a way that is meaningful to every provider.

We call the third type of information *creative information,* which we define as information used for the purpose of producing something or dealing with uncertainty (e.g., a recipe being used to bake a great cake or how to best care for a patient with pneumonia). For a physician, as well as other members of a patient's healthcare team, the standard is often the clinical information contained in an evidence-based guideline. The literature is replete with recommendations on how to incorporate evidence-based content directly in the EHR as a necessary initiative to reduce variability, quickly translate knowledge into orders, and improve patient outcomes. VBC has steadily become the cornerstone reimbursement methodology to change provider behavior from transaction-based care to longitudinal patient-centered care. With CMS' Primary Care First Model initiative launched in 2021, CMS is aggressively moving the market toward value-based payment, and commercial payers are keeping a steady pace. All of these payers are striving toward a common aim: reforming how healthcare is delivered and paid for to better care for individuals, provide better health for populations, and lower costs by shifting payment methodologies to paying providers based on the quality rather than the quantity of care provided. Payers have used a myriad of tools aimed at controlling overutilization of services that are not cost-effective and have experimented with various methods to monetize value to determine which yields the highest return (think of the hospital readmission reduction program or bundled payments). Hospital executives, however, haven't been as aggressive as the payers, and practice behaviors that may compromise the community, the hospital, and the patients remain the status quo.

Reinforcing the Power of Evidence-Based Protocols

The one VBC strategy that has withstood the test of time is the combination of objective, empirical evidence and subjective medical judgment in the form of evidence-based protocols (Health Research & Educational Trust, 2013; McCombs, 2019). Under many of the new VBC models, providers are incentivized to use evidence-based medicine, which is often referred to as the gold standard of care. In a new and evolving healthcare market that rewards efficiency, quality, and low costs, hospital leaders are looking to reduce variations in care to generate better results for patients and more savings for their organizations. One way to accomplish this is by focusing on evidence-based care protocols: the clinical care recommendations supported by the best available evidence in the clinical literature. And in hospitals, evidence-based medicine generally translates into the use of protocols, standardized order sets, practice flow charts, or, more recently, clinical decision support tools embedded in electronic medical records that work seamlessly in the background.

Physicians are barraged with a vast volume of new information, and it's difficult for them to stay abreast of all current research findings. Protocols are practice plans for the management of a clinical situation or process of care that will apply to most patients. They are not intended to replace individual clinical judgment but offer evidence-based structure when developing a patient's care plan. Protocols, rather than dictating a one-size-fits-all approach to patient care, provide recommendations that are based on a systematic review of evidence. They are generally developed through group consensus within a medical/surgical department or in combination with faculty within an academic medical center.

The Institute of Medicine (now the National Academy of Medicine) has been studying guidelines for over 30 years, with their first report on guidelines going back to 1990. Since then, the trustworthiness of the research behind protocols and the complexity of the first-generation formats have greatly improved for easier access and broader applicability in hospitals. Initially published as complicated free-text if-then statements that were inaccessible at the point of care, they have evolved into flowcharts, decision trees, and algorithms. Assisted by AI, "smart" treatment alternatives for the physician to consider are being integrated into the EHR based on the physician's clinical documentation. It is anticipated that once these smart EHRs start appearing in hospitals, they will improve clinical decision-making in a much more timely fashion.

The literature is replete with evidence of support and rejection of guidelines. Some physicians see them as helpful reminders for assimilating and locating information. Many supporters view guidelines as "encouraging interventions of proven benefit and discouraging the use of ineffective or potentially harmful interventions" (Murad, 2017). Others argue that the content of some guidelines are of questionable validity, the complexity of choices do not represent the experienced clinician's thought processes, and the choices of treatment options make them impractical to use during the care of a patient. Alternatively, some argue that the movement to simplify formats does not adequately account for all the factors present in patient care experience nor can they be used in the absence of information specific to the patient being treated.

Much of the resistance can also be traced to generational differences. One of us attended a conference several years ago and heard anecdotes from Dr. Brent James, former executive director of the Institute for Health Care Delivery Research. Known internationally for his work in clinical quality improvement, Dr. James described early medical practice as a cottage industry where physicians brought all their medical school, residency training, CME courses, journal reading, and clinical experience to the bedside to reach an individualized clinical decision (Swensen et al., 2010). These Boomers and GenXers "hand-crafted" a treatment plan that would be highly variable since no two physicians share exactly the same training and experience.

Dr. James' observations also confirm Dr. John Wennberg's pioneering work in the practice of medicine that proved that much of clinical medical practice across the United States remains empirical characterized by wide geographic variations that have no basis in clinical science. Dr. Wennberg was the first to study patterns of healthcare usage as well as variations in health cost and outcomes. Among his early research findings was a disturbing discrepancy in healthcare resource utilization among different geographic areas. In 1969, as the director of Vermont's new regional medical program, Dr. Wennberg found that resource utilization for a single procedure code differed depending upon ZIP code location. According to Gale (2016), "at that time he discovered that children (including his own) living in Waterbury Center, Vermont, had a 20% rate of having their tonsils removed. In the adjacent town of Stowe, the tonsillectomy rate was 60%. This threefold geographical difference in surgical procedures had a major impact on Wennberg and formed the basis for his subsequent research over the next forty-plus years."

He applied the same data analysis to other states and discovered that a similar pattern of geographic variations occurs across the country. Another example is a study of the percentage of people with dementia who have feeding tubes. The findings varied from a low of 1.3% in Portland, Oregon, to 14% in Lake Charles, Louisiana. Furthermore, he discovered that higher resource spending was not associated with improved outcomes. At a lecture one author of this book attended at Dartmouth University in New Hampshire, Dr. Wennberg produced research intended to explain the wide variations and concluded that geographic areas with a greater supply of healthcare services give more, often unnecessary, care and that physicians practice differently depending on where they live rather than based on the latest research. His conclusion has been confirmed in many published studies. One, by Hlatky and DeMara (2013), reported that when "standards of care in medicine are clear, practice patterns are similar in every part of the country. When there is no clear evidence on the best practices, however, different physicians will adopt different approaches, on the basis of their beliefs, training, incentives, and the local 'practice style'." The literature on practice variations is vast, and healthcare providers and policymakers are increasingly aware of the U.S. healthcare spending problem brought on by these practice patterns. Patients are also learning that more is not always better when it comes to medical tests and procedures.

Younger physicians recognize that medicine is changing so quickly that no single physician can stay current on any single area of medicine (Jacobson and Woloff, 2009). Millennial physicians, who comprise the majority of hospitalists (Martin, 2020), are more team-based and technologically savvy and want to make sure that they are equipped with as much knowledge as possible as they enter the patient's room. Clinical practice guidelines are natural tools to them because teams of multiple medical experts have come together to provide a road map for care of the patient. Where some physicians will try to avoid guidelines, using pejorative terms like "cookbook medicine," the younger, incoming generation, raised on the internet and technologically savvy, will embrace them much more easily and find that they improve care.

In 2001, the Institute of Medicine released a landmark report entitled *Crossing the Quality Chasm: A New Health System for the 21st Century,* which was essentially a follow-up to the now infamous 1999 Institute of Medicine report that took the United States healthcare system to task on one urgent quality problem: patient safety. In its earlier report, *To Err is Human: Building a Safer Health System,* the Institute concluded that tens of thousands of Americans die each year from errors in their care, and that hundreds of thousands more suffer or barely escape from nonfatal medical mistakes that a truly high-quality care system would largely prevent. The patient safety report was a call for action to make healthcare safer, and one can see the impact today, as all of the major healthcare accrediting organizations now include specific standards designed to improve patient safety at all sites of care. With the shift toward VBC, there is the potential to use enterprisewide surveillance with interdisciplinary care plans for conditions like sepsis, although this approach is not currently prevalent.

Unfortunately, adoption of protocols is not universal, and Luciano, Aloia, and Brett (2019) report that "attempting to 'plug in' a new practice often conflicts with the prevailing culture and existing practices and meets resistance from care providers. But deviating from the evidence-base can weaken the effectiveness of the practice and lessen the benefits."

Closing Comments From Stefani Daniels, RN

Back in 1984, the American College of Physicians wrote in a position paper, "Now and in the future under Medicare prospective payment, there are different needs for a form of utilization review. For example, in order for hospitals to deliver services most efficiently, it will be necessary for hospitals to review the service delivery, and for PROs (precursor to QIO) to monitor both over- and under-utilization." The report went on to say, "In addition, for those patients not covered by Medicare and continue to be covered by cost- or charge-based reimbursement, the payers themselves will wish to be assured that service utilization is as efficient as possible. The College supports UR mechanisms as a means of controlling health care costs and believes that greater efficiency in the use of resources is an appropriate means of reducing costs."

The authors of this position paper couldn't have imagined that the issues they identified in 1984 would still be present in 2021. Nor could they have imagined the persistent and unconscionable absence of any serious resource utilization monitoring. Yet, here we are today, facing similar pressures from Medicare, increasing demands from commercial payers, and a population frustrated with our entire healthcare system.

When confronted with unusual environmental transformations, successful organizations grab on to new challenges and new opportunities and adopt a change-ready culture to maintain its status among peers. But unlike any other American industry, hospitals have a dual governance structure that has a direct influence on management's ability to operate as efficiently or react to environmental pressures as rapidly as its corporate cousins. Whether nonprofit or for-profit, the administrative structure runs parallel to the medical staff structure. This dual governance arrangement has largely been responsible for hospitals' failure to operationally advance and financially thrive. Having spent most of my career in the executive suite of hospitals, I know that unless operational improvements are endorsed and actively supported by the more influential medical staff members, hospital executives will try to slowly maneuver needed changes to lessen medical staff resistance and physician threats "to take my patients elsewhere." In 2018, 21 hospitals closed, 47 closed in 2019, and 20 closed in 2020 (Ellison, 2020). There are probably many contributing factors that forced these closures, including strategies used by the payers to steer patients to lower-cost outpatient providers, such as the recent UnitedHealthcare policy decision to deny payment for nonemergent emergency department (ED) services—which, as previously mentioned, has been postponed due to the ongoing COVID-19 pandemic and the legal implications given Emergency Medical Treatment and Active Labor Act requirements. Nevertheless, UnitedHealthcare's intent is clear, and hospital executives should heed the warning and work with the medical staff to design new processes in anticipation of more strategies to deny hospital payment. For decades, hospital executives have closed their eyes to the inevitable, but unless cost reduction strategies and quality of care initiatives are implemented and endorsed by the medical staff—initiatives like evidence-based practice guidelines—hospitals will continue to face financial challenges and closures will continue, depriving communities of a much-needed resource.

There are some notable exceptions, such as Kaiser Permanente and Cleveland Clinic, both of which have had a salaried physician model for decades. As such, physicians are incentivized to cooperate for a common good, to collaborate with administration to identify opportunities to improve quality of care and to use resources wisely. They don't get paid for doing more—they get paid for doing well. Shared values are what separates Kaiser and Cleveland Clinic from the typical hospital and why they are consistently featured on the best hospital reports. Today, hospital executives have similar cooperation opportunities through the growth of hospitalist employment. Whether a contractual service provided by a local/regional physician group or a model of individual employment contracts, the C-suite has the opportunity to contractually address many of the quality and cost expectations for the practicing physician. I certainly hope they see the value in that approach. The status quo is not an option.

This entire book is replete with activities that are designed to compensate for the failure of the medical staff to cooperate with administration and comply with basic requirements that contribute to hospital survival: Knowledge of and adhering to rules and regulations that govern hospital operations and economic well-being; documenting their patient's story in a manner that makes sense to all readers today and in the future; and avoiding patient exposure to iatrogenic risk through misuse, underuse, or excessive use of resources. It's not entirely the physicians' fault: They are not taught how to work in a hospital, and many believe they shouldn't be concerned about the administrative and financial implications of providing care. But as new physicians educated and trained according to new standards and in a new environment enter the workforce, as outpatient care replaces the demand for inpatient care, as disparities in access to care and the exorbitant costs of care become untenable, the healthcare industry in general, and hospitals in particular, will have to change course.

Closing Comments From Ronald Hirsch, MD

When I started medical school back in 1984, I never envisioned where I would be in 2021. In fact, the concept of a new millennium seemed so far away. My residency was at Kaiser Permanente Medical Center in Los Angeles, one of the first integrated healthcare delivery systems in the country. However, in my three years there, I had little training in UR, other than assisting in transferring Kaiser patients back into the system when they were hospitalized at outside facilities. I entered private practice in 1991 in the Chicago area and joined the medical staff at two local community hospitals. Back then, there were no hospitalists: I saw my patients in the office and rounded at the hospital both before and after office hours. I took calls 24 hours a day from my own patients but shared weekend coverage with my partners. I vaguely recall being shown my length-of-stay data by the chief medical officer once. I think I was an outlier, but I justified it because my patients were sicker than all the other doctors' patients.

In 2006, I was asked to consider applying for the job of physician advisor (PA). I had no idea what that was, but I enjoyed interacting with the "discharge planners" at the hospital and thought it sounded intriguing. I had a short orientation from a consulting company and was then told to go out and be a PA, whatever that meant. I dug up some articles and found an online discussion forum and a case management professional society and joined both. I did my best to read and understand Medicare regulations. I yelled at my share of payer medical directors when they denied our admissions. I stalked the ED, trying to prevent avoidable admissions.

As time went by, I learned the nuances of the job. I developed relationships with my case managers, the hospital medical staff, the administration, and the board of directors. I learned to balance the needs of the hospital, the doctors, and most importantly, the patients. I started to understand hospital operations. I dug into the nuances of finance. I started speaking at conferences. I was never shy about speaking up on Medicare and contractor phone calls and, as a result, developed a reputation, good to some and bad to others.

In 2012, I left my comfort zone and took a job with a national company that provides compliance and revenue cycle services to hospitals. With this job, I was able to expand my knowledge and my perspective. And the first thing I learned was that some of the things we were doing at my hospital were wrong. Like many others, we were getting an order for observation after the standard surgery recovery period of four to six hours, and of course after reading this book, you know that is wrong.

I also discovered things are very different at other institutions. Most PAs and UR staff know their medical staff with their nuances and quirks. Now multiply that times 5,000 hospitals, and you can see how the number of permutations is staggering. Even today, I get questions from around the country that suggest a lot of people are still doing things wrong. What I determined was that many UR professionals and PAs learn their job from their coworkers and rarely are the regulations actually read. That's why I was excited to be able to coauthor this book, to try to be sure the right information got to the right people at the right time.

I have also realized that the vast majority of physicians and hospital administrators want to do the right thing. But since I started reading the daily news briefs from the Office of Inspector General, I realized that a small number don't, and because of their behavior, all of us must face increased scrutiny and seemingly endless audits. I will admit though, at my hospital there were a few doctors whose motives were other than noble. So, if my 250-bed suburban community hospital had a few, I suspect every hospital has the same. These few took up an inordinate amount of my time, be it reviewing their admissions, defending their admissions to insurance companies, and contacting them to find out why their patient remained in the hospital. I think knowing the rules is important to ensure that patients are getting the right care in the right setting.

But I did not ignore the other doctors. There was no way to expect even the best and brightest physicians to keep up with the regulatory changes. That was not why they became doctors, so I attended department meetings, wrote newsletters and personal letters, spent time in the doctor's lounge, and educated doctors of all specialties. Now I can do all of that on a much larger scale, both with my work with our clients and with the professional societies, and of course with this book.

As Stefani discussed, the Dartmouth Atlas data has shown there is great variation in the practice of medicine around the country. I would go one step further and say there is great variation even within states and within hospitals. I can still remember discussing a patient with a recent cardiac stent who was hospitalized with a gastrointestinal bleed. I asked the hospitalist about resuming aspirin and what he thought of an article that had recently been published in a major medical journal demonstrating the safety of resumption of aspirin at discharge. He told me, "I am too busy to have time to read journals." I spoke with a urologist who practiced in a smaller town in the Midwest about status determinations for patients having transurethral resection of the prostate. He keeps all his patients two days after surgery and was amazed to learn that there are doctors who routinely discharge their patients the next day, and even some who discharge the same day. He had no idea that the practice had changed since he left training or that the hospital did not get paid extra for those two days his patients remained in the hospital. In fact, as I was writing this section, the American Heart Association released a position statement entitled, "Evidence-Based Practices in the Cardiac Catheterization Laboratory" (Bangalore, 2021). In this paper, they address many dogmas that have persisted despite a paucity of evidence supporting them, such as "NPO after midnight," premedicating patients with shellfish allergy prior to angiography, and holding metformin for 48 hours prior to angiography. It is long past time for evidence to overrule dogma.

Hospital UR is not the sexiest job. You will never see a "Top 10 UR Specialists in America" list in *US News and World Report* as you do with orthopedic surgeons. But that does not diminish the importance of the role. The provision of medical care around the world has undergone unexpected and drastic changes during the COVID-19 pandemic, and the evolution of our healthcare system is unlikely to ever end. Whether "value" replaces "volume" as the predominant means of reimbursement is yet to be seen, but what is clear is that there will be change. I personally do not think we have yet figured out how to properly measure value and worry that the shift will result in unintended adverse consequences, as it did in the 1990s with the rapid growth of HMOs. In fact, I tease that ACOs are not new, we simply changed the way we spell HMO. So, as our healthcare system changes, I want our medical professionals to be able to dedicate their time and efforts to keeping up with the many advances in medical care and my colleagues in UR to keep up with the changes in the rules and regulations. Together I am confident that we can provide better care to more patients.

References

Bangalore, S., et al., on behalf of the American Heart Association Interventional Cardiovascular Care Committee of the Council on Clinical Cardiology; Council on Arteriosclerosis. (30 June 2021). Evidence-Based Practices in the Cardiac Catheterization Laboratory: A Scientific Statement from the American Heart Association. *Circulation, 144*(5). Retrieved from *https://www.ahajournals.org/doi/10.1161/ CIR.0000000000000996.*

Ellison, A. (December 2020). 21 hospital closures in 2020. Retrieved from *https://www. beckershospitalreview.com/finance/21-hospital-closures-in-2020.html.*

Gale, A. (2016). John Wennberg, MD: The Influential Doctor Who Blames Physicians and Fee-For-Service Medicine for the High Cost of Health Care. Obama Care is Based on His Research. *Missouri Medicine, 113*(3):156–158.

Health Research & Educational Trust. (April 2013). Metrics for the Second Curve of Health CareChicago, IL. Retrieved from *www.hpoe.org.*

Hlatky, M. A., and DeMaria, A. N. (2013). Does Practice Variation Matter? *Journal of the American College of Cardiology, 62*(5):447–448. Retrieved from *https://www.jacc.org/doi/full/10.1016/j.jacc.2013.05.013.*

Holt, M. (12 October 2020). Value-based care – No progress since 1997? The Health Care Blog. Retrieved from *https://thehealthcareblog.com/blog/category/health-policy/value-based-care/.*

Jacobson, J. O., and Wolff, A. C. (2009). Evidence-Based Medicine: Do Clinical Practice Guidelines Contribute to Better Patient Care? An Expert Interview With Drs. Joseph O. Jacobson and Antonio C. Wolff. Medscape. Retrieved from *https://www.medscape.org/viewarticle/589088.*